Prefix
MTW

0101315

KT-143-029

Genito-Urinary Medicine for Nurses

Genito-Urinary Medicine for Nurses

Alison Sutton and Stephanie Payne

Whurr Publishers Ltd
London

© 1996 Whurr Publishers Ltd
First published 1996 by
Whurr Publishers Ltd
19b Compton Terrace, London N1 2UN, England

Reprinted 1997

All rights reserved. No part of this publication may be
reproduced, stored in a retrieval system, or transmitted in
any form or by any means, electronic, mechanical, photo-
copying, recording or otherwise, without the prior
permission of Whurr Publishers Limited.

This publication is sold subject to the conditions that it
shall not, by way of trade or otherwise, be lent, resold,
hired out, or otherwise circulated without the publisher's
prior consent in any form of binding or cover other than
that in which it is published and without a similar condition including this condition being imposed upon any
subsequent purchaser.

British Library Cataloguing in Publication Data
A catalogue record for this book is available from the
British Library.

ISBN 1 86156 011 7

UR 9701364

WJ
100.1

990072

THE LIBRARY
KENT & SUSSEX HOSPITAL
TUNBRIDGE WELLS
KENT TN4 8AT

Printed and bound in the UK by Athenaeum Press Ltd,
Gateshead, Tyne & Wear.

Contents

Contributors

Maureen BAKER (RGN, SCM, FPC, Radiotherapy Cert.) Sister, Department of GU Medicine, Dewi Sant Hospital, Pontypridd.

Nicola CHURCH (RGN) Staff Nurse, Department of GU Medicine, Guest Hospital, Dudley at time of writing. Presently HIV Advisor, Health Promotion, Dudley.

Bernice FAGAN (RGN) Sister, The Ambrose King Centre, The Royal London Hospital, London.

Malcolm GOWARDUN (RGN, Cert. in Education) Charge Nurse, The Patrick Clements Clinic, Central Middlesex Hospital, London.

Jean HALE (RGN, RFN, FPC, AMIP) Senior Clinical Nurse Manager, Department of GU Medicine, Royal Gwent Hospital, Newport.

Pauline HANDY (RGN, FETC) Senior Staff Nurse, Department of GU Medicine, Newcastle General Hospital, Newcastle.

Paul HUSBAND (RGN, RMN, ONC) Charge Nurse, Milne Centre, Department of GU Medicine, Bristol Royal Infirmary, Bristol.

Sue MANSELL (RGN) Specialty Manager, Department of GU Medicine, Royal Hospital, Wolverhampton.

Gabrielle MCDERMOTT (RGN) Sister, Department of GU Medicine, Withington Hospital, Manchester.

Christina MCGLYNN (RGN) Sister, The Ambrose King Centre, The Royal London Hospital, London.

Sally-Ann PALMER (RGN) Sister, Department of GU Medicine, Royal Bournemouth General Hospital, Bournemouth.

Stephanie PAYNE (RGN) Sister, Department of GU Medicine, Royal Hospital, Wolverhampton at time of writing. Presently Sister, Marlborough Clinic, Royal Free Hospital, London.

Mary PHILLIPS (RGN) Senior Sister, The Ambrose King Centre, The Royal London Hospital, London.

Alison SUTTON (RGN) Sister, Department of GU Medicine, Guest Hospital, Dudley at time of writing. Presently HIV Liaison Nurse, Guest Hospital, Dudley.

Preface

Very few books are available in nursing libraries that relate to Genito-Urinary Medicine (GUM) nursing. As nurses working in this field of nursing, we felt this lack should be remedied. This book on genito-urinary (GU) nursing has been written specifically for GU nurses by GU nurses. It contains important information for nursing students with an interest in sexual health matters and other nurses working in related sexual health areas, such as family planning.

We have concentrated on what actually happens in a GUM department and the role of the nurse. Since the advent of HIV/AIDS, *The Scope of Professional Practice* (UKCC, 1992) and the formation of the Genito-Urinary Nurses Association (GUNA) in 1991, nurses working in GUM departments have gained a higher profile.

This book will be a valuable resource for all GUM departments. It gives a general overview of GU nursing to those new to the specialty and consolidates past experiences of GU nurses around the country, to enable them to write clinical practices and standards for nursing care in their own departments. As a group of GU nurses from clinics around England and Wales, sharing information and first-hand experiences, we hope to improve the quality of care given to patients attending GUM.

This book proves that GUM is an up and coming area. Throughout the country, nurses have very different levels of responsibility in GUM clinics, along with different gradings, as has been shown in research published by Allen and Hogg (1993) and The Monks Report (1988).

Courses and education in this particular field have been sadly lacking over the years. Consequently, many GU nurses have found difficulty in gaining a place on a relevant course and then in keeping up-to-date. However, this is being rectified with the advent of PREP and the competition between colleges of nursing, linked to universities, offering more courses of interest in specialised areas. We hope this book will help stimulate nurses who are interested in furthering their education and thus their career, in this field of nursing.

Alison Sutton
Stephanie Payne
April, 1996

Acknowledgements

We are extremely grateful to Glaxo Wellcome UK, Roche Products Limited and the Royal Wolverhampton Hospitals NHS Trust for sponsoring this book. Without them it would not have been possible.

We would like to thank our families, Adrian, Katy and Tim, for their patience, love and support through many long weekends and nights and for keeping us going.

To our managers and colleagues at Wolverhampton, the Royal Free and Dudley hospitals, many thanks for your support, particularly to Barbara and Jane, medical librarians in Dudley. Many thanks also to Jim, the publishers and of course, to the contributors.

This book is dedicated to GUNA and all GUM nurses.

The views expressed in this publication are not necessarily those of the sponsors.

Table of Parliamentary Acts, Reports and Regulations

1864	The Contagious Diseases Act
1866	The Contagious Diseases Act
1869	The Contagious Diseases Act
1916	Final Report of the Royal Commission on Venereal Disease
1974	NHS Venereal Disease Regulations
1984	Data Protection Act
1990	Access to Public Records Act
1991	The National Health Service Trusts (Venereal Diseases) Directions
1992	Medicinal Products: Prescription by Nurses Act

Chapter 1
Genito-urinary nursing

Sue Mansell and Stephanie Payne

The Role of the Genito-urinary Nurse

Research has shown that the work carried out by nurses in genito-urinary medicine (GUM) clinics varies considerably from clinic to clinic (Rogers & Adler, 1987; The Monks Report, 1988; Allen & Hogg, 1993). This chapter aims to motivate nurses working in this specialty to improve their skills and develop good quality practice. Nurses have a responsibility to update themselves in the care and management of sexually transmitted infections in order to give patients the care and support they need. Since the advent of human immunodeficiency virus (HIV) infection and acquired immune deficiency syndrome (AIDS) and with the targets set in *The Health of the Nation* (DOH, 1993a), GUM has received a much higher profile; it is no longer considered to be a 'Cinderella service'. In-house study days relating to sexual health issues are being arranged locally for nurses and the ENB course 276 'Caring for people with sexually transmitted infections' is becoming more accessible nationwide. GU nurses around the country have joined together to form their own association, The Genito-Urinary Nurses Association (GUNA), which provides twice-yearly updates, newsletters and guidelines specifically related to GU nursing.

The multidisciplinary team

In GUM, nurses may work with doctors, health advisers, technicians, clerical staff, psychologists, social workers, dietitians and other professionals, depending on the size and locality of the clinic, thus making up a multidisciplinary team. Collectively, the staff have to be able to work together in harmony. Their roles and responsibilities vary from clinic to clinic for different reasons, as demonstrated by Allen & Hogg (1993). Work carried out by GU nurses will often overlap with that of their colleagues because the team works so closely together. It is important to acknowledge one's limitations, to liaise with other members of the multidisciplinary team and refer patients to them as appropriate. As patients may discuss very personal issues with a doctor, a nurse and a health adviser, it is imperative that staff complement each other in all they say and do.

Everyone wants their clinic to give a good impression to the patient, especially in this time of purchaser/provider negotiations and service contracts. Good staff support and efficient communication systems need to be in place to promote a good working environment for staff. This, in turn, enables staff to create a caring environment for patients. Providing effective, high quality care to a patient attending a GUM clinic can only be achieved when the multidisciplinary team share the same standards of care and expectations. As in any other sphere of health care, the quality of the service has to be measured by having monitoring and audit systems in place. Clinical audit is now taking place in GUM clinics throughout Britain and, if well documented, will give a research base for good practice as quality, outcomes and audit was an area in which targets for action were set in *A Vision for the Future* (DOH, 1993b). All staff working in the GUM clinic must be encouraged to participate in standard-setting so that the standards are owned collectively and reach their maximum potential. Clinic protocols and standards of care have to be developed amongst the team so that all the staff agree. This helps to form a philosophy for the GUM department and enables everyone to strive towards common goals for the good of patients.

Regular staff meetings, making sure that each discipline is represented, will provide an arena for information to be disseminated and any problems to be discussed. For reference, records of each meeting should be kept so that people who are unable to attend can keep up-to-date; verbal feedback is also crucial. It is important for staff to be appraised at least annually. Appraisals can help morale if carried out with genuine interest and can enable nurses to step forward. As well as showing a healthy interest in individuals and their wellbeing, time taken to reflect on an individual's work and review the current situation helps to ensure that the personal development and educational needs of all team members are met so that nurses can deliver high quality care.

Communication

It is essential that the GU nurse has good communication skills. As well as communicating with members of the multidisciplinary health care team to maintain the team spirit, the nurse's role encompasses educating and counselling patients. With the stigma that has been attached to GUM clinics in the past, it may seem a daunting prospect for a patient to attend a GUM department, especially for the first time when they have no idea what to expect. Individualised patient care has to be given as everyone's needs are different. Patients will display a range of different emotions. Initially patients often feel embarrassed about having to attend the department and may be very distressed, frightened or angry, depending on their reason for attending. As talking about sexual matters is an extremely sensitive issue, it is of paramount importance that attention is paid to the provision of an appropriate environment and adequate privacy. Simple things like making sure that the door to a room is closed properly and having an 'engaged' sign on the door will help to put patients more at ease. Patients must be allowed the time they need to be able to talk and so that they can take in the information they are given. Some patients will ask more questions and take up more time than others. The patient must be prepared for what is going to happen before any tests or treatments are carried out. Nurses should ensure that the patient has understood what the doctor has said to them during their initial interview and give a clear, concise explanation of what is to follow. Appropriate language and terminology should be used, even slang where necessary (Adler, 1990), so that patients can more easily understand what is going on. Medical jargon and abbreviations should be avoided and listening skills developed. Patients will often tell nurses things that they have omitted to tell the receptionist when registering at the clinic or the doctor whilst being interviewed. Some people just want someone to listen to them, as they have no one else to turn to or feel unable to confide in anyone outside the clinic. Many people find it difficult to talk about their sexuality and sexual health matters and this problem is often enhanced for lesbians and gay men as they may have extra stress when using health care services because of the possibility of homophobia (James, Harding & Corbett, 1994).

Attitudes

The Code of Professional Conduct (UKCC, 1992a), which all registered nurses are required to work to, states that nurses must:

recognise and respect the uniqueness and dignity of each patient and client, and respond to their need for care, irrespective of their ethnic origin, religious beliefs, personal attributes, the nature of their health problems or any other factor.

It is important to remember this in GUM and maintain a non-judgmental attitude towards patients when it comes to matters of sexuality and sexual practices. Moral and sexual attitudes may differ, but this has to be accepted in order to be able to care for patients properly (Adler, 1990). As in any other field of medicine, nurses are not there to inflict their views and morals on others, but to reliably inform and educate patients so that they are empowered to make informed decisions about their lifestyles, thus promoting health. Nurses are there to support patients, no matter who they are or what they do. GU nursing can be quite stressful for nurses if they feel uncomfortable about dealing with people who might be described as promiscuous, gay, drug users or sex workers. Such people do make up a proportion of GUM patients and can challenge the religious, personal and cultural ideals held by nurses (Palmer, 1995). Nurses have to withhold their prejudices and not show signs of disapproval. They are not there to induce feelings of guilt or to apportion blame. Adler (1990) states that 'it is bad manners for staff to force their own attitudes on a patient and it is also bad medicine, since the patient will not come back'. It is better that sympathy and understanding is shown to patients with sexual health problems to make the most of an opportunity for giving information and advice appropriate to the patient's behaviour. This will then add to the strategy for preventing sexually transmitted diseases (STDs) (Adimora et al., 1994).

Named nurse initiative

According to *The Patient's Charter* (DOH, 1992) every patient or client should have a named nurse (a registered nurse who is responsible for the care that a patient receives). This often results in more personal recognition and satisfaction for the patient and for the nurse.

GU nurses work in an ideal climate for implementing the named nurse initiative. It works particularly well if the same nurse can deal with the same patient throughout his or her visit to the clinic. Continuity of care is maintained if one nurse assesses the patient, performs the tests and administers the treatment and there is further benefit if the same nurse can see the patient on their follow-up visit to evaluate the care given. The quality of care is enhanced by the nurse being able to build up a rapport with the patient and there is a better chance of the patient complying with treatment. This ensures the delivery of high quality, cost effective care and helps staff to meet the first target in *A Vision for the Future* (DOH, 1993b) concerning individualised patient care. In order to monitor the quality and effectiveness of care given to patients, nurses must ensure that their work is accurately and clearly documented.

Documentation

Continuity of individualised care will be promoted by good record-keeping as this is an effective means of communicating information to all members of the team providing care for a patient (UKCC, 1993). A set of records is made for each patient on registration at a GUM clinic; they are totally confidential and are not held with the general hospital records. The records are usually collaborative and every discipline working in GUM is responsible for recording information in the patients' notes at one time or another. In line with the *Standards for Records and Record-keeping* (UKCC, 1993), nurses must ensure that they write in black ink and that all entries are signed and dated. To help maintain high standards of care and avoid errors, nurses must make sure that they have signed to say what treatments or tests have been given or carried out and report on the patient's progress. This will also help in maintaining the named nurse protocol as other members of the team can see at a glance which nurse is responsible for the patient's care.

Heywood Jones (1989) identifies that 'maintaining good records is an important part of every practitioner's work'. Meticulous record-keeping benefits staff as well as patients, especially in litigation cases. Any document which records any aspect of the care of a patient can be required as evidence before a court of law or before the Professional Conduct Committee of the UKCC or other similar regulatory bodies for the health care professions (UKCC, 1993). The patient's case notes can provide a lasting record of what has been observed or done, demonstrate the chronology of events and state the clinical decisions made relating to patient care (UKCC, 1993). Also, records might help serious, perhaps lethal, errors from being made, for example, in relation to drug administration. All nurses have a responsibility and a legal duty for the safe-keeping of patients' notes so that all information remains confidential.

Confidentiality

A separate set of patient records is created and stored in the GUM department to comply with *The National Health Service Trusts*

(Venereal Diseases) Directions 1991. The confidentiality principle is explained to all new patients. Some clinics ask patients to sign a consent form allowing them to disclose information only in accordance with these Directions. Other clinics use a consent form relating to cytology and colposcopy results and follow-up. This is to ensure that true, informed consent is obtained from the patient before examination or treatment begins.

The registration number given to the patient on his or her first attendance at the GUM department bears no relation to his or her hospital number. The importance of retaining the GUM number is carefully explained to each patient to help maintain confidentiality. This number is used on any specimens or forms that leave the department instead of giving the patient's name, thus preserving their anonymity.

Confidentiality is of prime importance in this area of patient care: patients would be less likely to attend the GUM department if they thought that information given was not going to be kept confidential. Also, one must remember the difficulties faced by some people who have been tested for HIV in relation to getting a mortgage or life insurance. In a survey of 520 patients considering having HIV tests in GUM clinics, over 25% said that when applying for life insurance they would probably lie about ever having had a test (Hulme, Smith & Barton, 1992).

Any information capable of identifying an individual who is attending the GUM department must be kept locked away when the department is left unattended and then shredded or incinerated when it is time for disposal.

The Patient's Charter, Right Six (DOH, 1992), relays to patients that they can have access to their health records and know that those working for the NHS are under a legal duty to keep their contents confidential. This is derived from the specific statutory duty imposed by the *1990 Access to Health Records Act* which follows on from the *1984 Data Protection Act* which gave patients access to their computerised records (Friend, 1992). Patients have to go through the system of applying for access to the records held about them in the GUM department, as they would for their general case notes held in the hospital's medical records department. Access to information that would identify a third party is not allowed to be revealed. Therefore, records made by the health adviser are not accessible because information relating to their sexual contacts may be recorded there.

If health care staff are to meet the targets set in *The Health of the Nation* document (DOH, 1993a) concerning the reduction of gonorrhoea and teenage pregnancies, it is imperative that young people under the age of 16 are assured of confidentiality. 'The duty of confidentiality owed to a person under 16 is as great as that owed to any other person' (British Medical Association et al., undated).

Nurse-led Services

Understanding of nurse-run clinics varies from clinic to clinic. It may be that nurses run a particular clinic without medical staff being present (Allen & Hogg, 1993) or a nurse clinic may be in progress alongside a traditional clinic where medical staff are available if necessary. However, it is clear that in some GUM clinics certain activities are performed by doctors while in other clinics the same activity is carried out by nurses. The role of the GU nurse is often dictated by the clinic consultant or by clinic policy (Allen & Hogg, 1993).

Before 1992, some GU nurses held 'extended roles' – activities that were normally undertaken by the doctor were delegated in appropriate circumstances and performed by nurses who had received appropriate training (DHSS, 1989). Extended roles of some nurses included microscopy, cryotherapy, venepuncture and examination of a female patient (Allen & Hogg, 1993). Nurses needed to be specifically trained and had to prove competency for the given tasks. A certificate of competency was then issued. The delegating doctor also had to be assured of the competence of the nurse as he or she may have had some legal responsibility if anything went wrong.

The Extending Role of the Nurse document (DHSS, 1989) has now been superseded by *The Scope of Professional Practice*, (UKCC, 1992b). This means that each practitioner is subject to the *Code of Professional Conduct* (UKCC, 1992a) and is accountable for his or her practice and conduct. Extending the nurse's role is no longer deemed a suitable expression as this can limit practice rather than extend or expand it (UKCC, 1992b).

It is the Council's principles for practice, as set out in *The Scope of Professional Practice* (UKCC, 1992b) paragraphs 8–11 inclusive, that should form the basis for adjustments to the scope of practice, rather than having certificates for tasks. However, it is recognised that some mechanism should be in place to assess the competency of a practitioner. *The Scope of Professional Practice* (UKCC, 1992b) is about nurses taking the initiative, based on knowledge, skill and experience in order to improve their practice for the benefit of the patient. It is also about being accountable for any action taken. Nurse-run clinics have their foundation in the light of this knowledge.

Nursing practice

The study carried out by Allen and Hogg (1993) into work roles in GUM highlighted activities that are or could be developed in nurse clinics. These activities are shown in Table 1.1.

Table 1.1: Activities to be developed in nurse-run clinics

- Cytology screening
- Serological tests for syphilis
- Hepatitis B vaccinations and post-vaccination titres
- Treatment of anogenital warts by cryotherapy, podophyllin or trichloroacetic acid
- Tests of cure for review patients
- Giving results of tests
- HIV counselling and venepuncture
- Patient education, information and advice
- Giving out condoms and emergency contraception

It is clear that as nurses seek to expand their roles in GUM clinics, the consultants need to appreciate and provide opportunities for their staff to be trained and to develop professionally in competencies to complement their own important roles. However, nurses must recognise their own limitations and their practice must be safe, ethical and research-based. Clinical practices, protocols and guidelines need to be ratified and followed; examples from the author's clinic are given throughout this chapter (Figures 1.1–1.11 and appendix), although it should be noted that these will differ between clinics. Standard guidelines to aid with the process of developing such protocols are available from GUNA (GUNA, 1995).

The nurse must accept personal accountability for any action taken. The scope of professional practice looks at nurses setting their own agendas, rather than having them set by other disciplines.

Castledine (1994) notes that the following activities do little if anything to enhance the scope of nursing practice:

1.   handed down medical tasks;
2.   following physicians' orders;
3.   specimen collection and laboratory work;
4.   assisting doctors with procedures.

As GU nurses are encouraged to take on tasks like venepuncture, cryotherapy, cytology, wart treatments and assisting with colposcopies and biopsies, it is clear that these will do little to enhance the scope of nursing practice, but it is a beginning. Nurses need to be well trained, well informed and to constantly update their skills in these activities. Also, nurses' responsibilities from clinic to clinic need to be standardised according to grading.

In Clause 1 of the *1992 Medicinal Products: Prescription by Nurses Act*, it states that registered nurses, midwives and health visitors are appropriate practitioners for prescribing prescription-only medicines. Any nurse who wishes to prescribe must accept personal responsibility for ensuring they fulfil their code of conduct and have received appropriate education. Competency must be assessed and recorded and made available to bona fide enquirers such as pharmacists (Andrews, 1994). Some hospitals have local multidiscipline protocols for those nurses who are competent to prescribe to follow.

It is clear that the role of the nurse is no longer seen as the handmaiden of the doctor. 'The unique role of GUM clinics in relation to the sexual health of the nation should be recognised' (Allen & Hogg, 1993). GU nurses need to be encouraged to extend the boundaries of their work to include giving appropriate contraceptive advice, so that the requirements identified in key area 4 of *The Health of the Nation* (DOH, 1993a) are met. Allen & Hogg (1993) identified the need for nurses to take every opportunity to give sex education and contraceptive advice, especially to young people and those clearly 'at risk' not only from infection but also from unwanted pregnancies.

In some clinics GU nurses have successfully developed their roles in health promotion, both inside and outside the clinic setting, for example, teaching within schools, colleges, youth hostels and youth clubs.

Kinnell (1993) identified that younger women were less likely than older women to attend clinics for STD screening or for contraceptive care and were more likely to be seriously misinformed about HIV transmission routes. The innovative initiatives of some GU nurses in taking the message of safe/safer sex out onto the streets, by using a 'condom-mobile' giving out free condoms and sexual health advice, may go some way to rectify this situation.

Nursing Care

A journey through the GUM clinic

Taking the aforementioned issues into consideration, the clinic staff can provide quality, holistic care to all who enter through the doors of GUM. People present at the clinic for many varied reasons. They

may have been asked to attend by their sexual partner, general practitioner (GP) or by another referral agency, for example, Victim
Support or Drug Care. Many patients refer themselves, either via a
telephone enquiry or by presenting at a clinic session. Most clinics in
Great Britain operate an appointment system, while some have
'walk-in' protocols and others run a combined system (see Figure 1.1).

A   Walk-in patients

    1   If appointment available
        Patient is to be seen

    2   If appointment NOT available
        Patient is to be offered first available appointment at a later clinic

        If patient still wishes to be seen at that session, they should be assessed by
        the health adviser/nurse in charge and, if deemed urgent, must be seen
        after discussion with the doctor

B   Request for 'urgent' appointment over the telephone
        Patient is to be advised to walk in to the clinic no later than 45 minutes
        before the end of the current session and told that they will be assessed
        by the health adviser/nurse in charge as detailed above

C   Patients arriving late for an appointment
        Patients who arrive more than 20 minutes late for their appointment will
        be seen at the discretion of the doctor

Figure 1.1: Protocol for walk-in patients
Reproduced with the kind permission of The Royal Wolverhampton Hospitals
NHS Trust.

The Monks Report (DOH, 1988) stated that all clinics should see
any person with a new clinical problem suggestive of an STD or who
considers himself or herself to have been in contact with such a
disease on the day of presentation or failing that on the next occasion
the clinic is open.

No two clinics function in the same way. The variable roles and
responsibilities of the nursing staff and the overlap of roles of the
different disciplines makes each clinic quite unique (Rogers & Adler,
1987). A useful way of understanding how a particular clinic runs is to
follow a new patient through all the stages of their appointment. That
is, registration, history taking, examination and tests, microscopy,
diagnosis, treatment and health advising interview. An example of the
progression through the clinic is demonstrated in Figure 1.2.

Even if the clinic is well staffed and efficiently run there will be
some waiting periods between each stage. These should be kept to a
minimum as they may aggravate any anxiety the patient already
feels. He or she may lose courage at any stage and disappear from

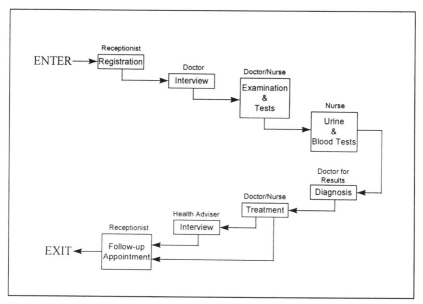

Figure 1.2: Flowchart of patients' progress through the clinic

the clinic. A patient may expect to be in the clinic for up to one and a half hours on their first visit so that all the necessary investigations can be completed.

Common presenting symptoms
A patient attending the clinic may or may not have symptoms. Arya, Osoba and Bennett (1988) note common presenting symptoms that indicate that a disease has or may have been sexually acquired and these are shown in Table 1.2. Nurses should bear in mind that a patient may be emotionally disturbed, especially if he or she has a history of mental, physical or sexual abuse.

Receiving a patient
The first contact a patient has with anyone in the GUM department is usually with the reception staff. The importance of this first contact must not be underestimated. At reception the assessment process begins. Whether consciously or unconsciously, a patient's verbal or non-verbal behaviour may reveal immediately the level of anxiety or distress he or she is experiencing. Patients demonstrating any depth of mental anguish should, if at all possible, be shown into the privacy of a room away from main reception. They should be seen immediately by the health adviser or nurse. Understanding and empathy displayed at this point, together with an explanation of procedures, can eliminate some initial apprehension.

Table 1.2: Common presenting symptoms

- Dysuria or genital discomfort
- Urethral discharge
- Genital ulceration
- Vaginal discharge
- Itching on or around genitalia
- Lower abdominal pain in women
- Painless swelling on genitalia or anus
- Discomfort on intercourse
- Scrotal pain or swelling
- Swelling in groin
- Ano-rectal symptoms (discharge, painful defecation)
- Skin rash
- Mucous membrane lesions
- Sore throat
- Eye lesions in the neonate

A warm, comfortable waiting room, with current magazines, health care literature and facilities for children helps to produce a good environment for waiting. Some clinics have background music, television and snack bar facilities.

Registration

The importance of confidentiality cannot be overemphasised. At the reception desk a new patient is asked to give personal details such as name, address, date of birth, occupation and name of family doctor. This information is obtained either verbally or in writing via a registration form and adequate privacy must be ensured. The registration form used in the authors' clinic is shown in Figure 1.3.

Most clinics keep either a manual register of patients in order of attendance or, more likely, patients' details are entered and stored on a computer database. If this method of storing demographic details of patients is used, patients must be made aware of this in line with the Data Protection Act 1984.

A registration number is allocated to the patient, and the importance of retaining this number is explained so that records can be located easily and to maintain confidentiality. An index card may be made out stating name, address, date of birth, registration number and date of registration and this should be stored in a lockable, alphabetical index filing system. This can help staff to find records more easily if the patient should forget their number.

PATIENT REGISTRATION FORM

We would be grateful if you could complete the form below to enable your details to be entered onto the computer. This information is protected under the Data Protection Act, 1984 and is extremely confidential. No information will be disclosed to anybody other than those working in this department providing you with health care. Please sign at the bottom of this form acknowledging that you have understood the above.

PLEASE PRINT CLEARLY AND CIRCLE THE APPROPRIATE ANSWER

1. Have you ever attended the clinic before?   Yes/No
    If yes, what is your clinic number: ....

2. Name ....Date of birth ....

3. Address ....

    ....

4. Postcode ....

5. Telephone number ....

6. What is your country of birth? ....

7. What is your ethnic origin? White/Black Caribbean/Black African/
        Black Other/Indian/Pakistani/Bangladeshi/Chinese/Other ethnic group

8. What is your occupation? ....

9. Who asked you to attend the clinic? ....

10. Are you Single/Married/Separated/Widowed/Divorced/Cohabiting?

11. Name of your family doctor ....

12. Address of your family doctor ....

    ....

Signature ....Date ....

Thank you. Please hand this form to the receptionist who will register you and give you a registration number and appointment card.

Figure 1.3: Patient registration form

Reproduced with the kind permission of The Royal Wolverhampton Hospitals NHS Trust.

A set of health records is created for the patient. When registration has been completed the patient is given an appointment card that bears their personal reference number and appropriate literature (i.e. information sheet or booklet). Guidelines for registering a new patient in the authors' clinic are shown in Figure 1.4.

History taking

In most clinics, the doctor is responsible for the initial interviewing of a patient. Good history taking is an art, learned through practice (Schofield, 1979). A complete, clear, concise history is often the key to a quick and accurate diagnosis. The patient may be prepared and anticipate some of the questions that the doctor may ask. Getting a patient to disclose personal intimate details of their sexual activity is a skilled task, in which confidentiality must be assured. It is helpful when collecting in-depth information to use a data-collecting tool like the one used in the authors' clinic and shown in Figure 1.5. By using an appropriate format, a method of questioning is developed by the interviewer. It may prove more productive to begin by focusing on less sensitive information, for example asking a patient about her menstrual history, rather than launching straight into questions about intimate sexual activity.

The clinical history is a guide to what investigations may be required. The types of sexual activity will indicate which areas of the body will require testing for infection. For example, if anal or oral sex have been reported, swabs from the rectum and throat may be taken.

Following the initial interview, the patient may be asked to wait before being called for physical examination. If a delay is anticipated, it is unwise to keep a patient waiting in an examination room as this environment may increase anxiety.

Examination and tests

Protocols for routine tests performed to detect sexually transmitted infections will vary from clinic to clinic and depend on the patient's history. The majority of patients attending GUM clinics are offered routine STD screening and this usually consists of tests for gonorrhoea, syphilis, *Trichomonas vaginalis*, chlamydia, candida and bacterial vaginosis. Some clinics routinely screen for mycoplasma and ureaplasma as well. For the results of these tests to be accurate the nurse has to be competent in collecting specimens from the genitalia,

RECEPTION AND REGISTRATION OF NEW PATIENTS

Information

In the department of genito-urinary medicine, we aim to establish a welcoming environment when the patient arrives for his/her appointment, and assure the patient of complete confidentiality

Equipment

Comfortable waiting room (with magazines, television, drinks machine and children's toys)
Request form for personal details
Pen
Information booklet
Appointment card
Folder, patient assessment sheet, evaluation sheet, results sheet and consent form
Computer terminal with access to printer
Adhesive labels
Index card

Action	Rationale
1 Welcome the patient on arrival to the clinic. Ascertain their name and previous clinic number (if they have attended before), and the time of their appointment	To receive the patient into the clinic quickly and efficiently, thus reducing the patient's stress level
2 Ask the patient to complete a request form for personal details. If he/she has difficulty in doing this, then the information should be sought verbally, ensuring that the patient has adequate privacy in which to do so. A nurse or health adviser may need to take the patient to a private room for this	To ensure confidentiality whilst obtaining the information required for the patient's case notes
3 If the patient has not attended the clinic before, give him/her an information booklet. Ask the patient to take a seat in the waiting room whilst you are entering his/her personal details on to the computer ensuring that the monitor screen is facing away from the reception area	To make the patient comfortable, and maintain confidentiality
4 When a registration number has been allocated to the patient, write it onto an appointment card and give it to the patient. Explain the importance of retaining this number in relation to maintaining confidentiality, and locating the patient's records more easily. Also, give the patient directions to the consulting rooms	To assure the patient about confidentiality, and orientate him/her re the layout of the clinic

Figure 1.4: Guidelines for reception and registration of new patients

5	Create a set of records for the patient, putting together a folder, a patient assessment sheet, an evaluation sheet, a results sheet and a consent form. Print out a copy of the patient's details from the computer and attach it to the front of the patient assessment sheet. Also, print out a set of labels for use on request forms and specimens, and staple these inside the front cover of the folder	To provide a record of the patient's details for all staff in the department to see
6	Carefully write the patient's registration number in black ink on the edge of the folder, unless the patient is already known to have had a positive syphilis test result, then write it in red ink. If the patient is known to be HIV positive, draw a red star by his/her number. If the patient is known to have been raped, put a red spot next to their number	To prepare the notes for numerical filing, and to identify records that have to be kept forever more easily. (This also helps to draw the attention of the doctor to a particular patient's condition)
7	Write out an index card stating the patient's name, address, date of birth, registration number and date of registration. Store in the alphabetical index filing system	To help in finding records more easily for patients who forget their number, and to provide an historical record

Bibliography

(for guidelines relating to receiving and registering new patients)
Adler MW (1990) ABC of Sexually Transmitted Diseases, 2nd edn. London: British Medical Association.
Catterall RD (1964) Venereology for Nurses. London: The English Universities Press Ltd.
Kinnersley P (1991) Recording information about new patients. Update 43(2).

Figure 1.4: *Continued*
Reproduced with the kind permission of The Royal Wolverhampton Hospitals NHS Trust.

urine testing and venepuncture. Specialist clinical practices for these procedures from the authors' clinic can be found in the appendix at the end of this chapter.

It is the nurse who usually prepares the patient for examination. All equipment needed should be collected before starting the tests. Swabs, slides, culture plates and bottles containing media need to be clearly labelled with the patient's GUM registration number and date of birth or date of examination, as dictated by clinic policy.

Date 1st Attend	THE ROYAL HOSPITAL WOLVERHAMPTON DEPARTMENT OF GENITO-URINARY MEDICINE		Registration No.	
Name:			Age:	DOB: / /
Address:			Civil State:	
Occupation:	Tel No.		Origin:	
Referred by:			Area:	
Name of G.P.			PENICILLIN ALLERGY	
Address of G.P.			YES	NO

History of Present Illness	Menstrual History
	L.M.P.
	Contraception
	Cytology

	Obstetric History: G: P
	   Live children
	   S.B.
	   Miscarriages
	   T.O.P.

Last Contact	
Contacts in past 3 months	Recent Drugs
Last Marital Contact	Smoking I.V.D.A.
	Alcohol
Past History of G.U. Infection	Sex Abroad
	Other Allergies
Past Medical History	Blood Transfusion
	Blood Donation
Family History	

Figure 1.5: Data collection tool

PHYSICAL EXAMINATION

Seen by: INVESTIGATIONS:

GENITAL EXAMINATION: FBC   ESR
Inguinal lymph nodes   VDRL
Labia   TPHA
Urethra   FTA (abs)   lg. G
Skene's ducts   Ig. M
Bartholin's glands
Vagina   URETHRAL SLIDE:
Vaginal discharge   Gc   Polys
Cervix   Epi   O.O.
Cervical discharge
Perineum   CERVICAL SLIDE:
Anus   Gc   Polys
Rectum   Epi   O.O.
Uterus   Chlamydia
Tubes
                                  RECTAL SLIDE
                                  Gc   Polys
                                  Epi   O.O.

GENERAL EXAMINATION:
                                  VAGINAL SLIDE:
Skin   Gc   TV
Mouth   Candida   Polys
Lymph nodes   GV   O.O.
Bones and Joints
C.V.S.B.P.   CULTURES:
                                  Urethral
R.S.   Cervical
Abdomen   Rectal
C.N.S.   Vaginal
                                    TV
                                    Candida
                                  Throat
                                  Chlamydia
                                  Mycoplasma
                                  Ureaplasma
                                  Bacteroids
                                  Viral
PROVISIONAL DIAGNOSIS: CERVICAL CYTOLOGY:

                                  URINE: P.U.   Hrs
                                  Protein
                                  Sugar
                                  Blood
                                  Ketones
TREATMENT: MSU

                                  D.G.
                                  DIFF QUICK

                                  PREGNANCY TEST:

                                  HIV ANTIBODIES:

CONTACT TRACING: HEPATITIS B ANTIBODY:

                                  X-RAYS:

                                  OTHER TESTS:

Figure 1.5: *Continued* Reproduced with the kind permission of The Royal Wolverhampton Hospitals NHS Trust.

The patient is shown into the examination room by the nurse. The nurse introduces himself or herself to the patient and explains what will happen, how long the procedure will take and why the procedure is necessary. The patient should be invited to ask questions. To undergo intimate questioning and examination can be extremely traumatic and an ordeal for any patient. Clinic staff need to be aware and sensitive to this fact, as this can affect the patient's ability to understand everything that they have been told. Patients may display emotional distress that can be projected onto the clinic personnel. It is important for staff to understand these situations and be adequately prepared.

Female examination

The patient is asked to remove any undergarments, tights or trousers so that the genital area can be examined. She is placed in the lithotomy position. If this is not possible, or if the patient prefers, a lateral position with the knees flexed and pointing outwards and heels together can be adopted. A good light source is needed.

The abdomen may be inspected noting size, contour and symmetry. Any abnormalities, for example, rash, scars, hernia or lesions need to be documented. Percussion and light or deep palpation of all quadrants of the abdomen may be performed if the patient's history suggests that this is necessary. Breasts may also be examined noting any lesions, rash, tenderness or swelling.

Inspection and palpation of the genital tract then takes place. See Figure 1.6 for the anatomy of the female genito-urinary tract. The skin over the vulva, perineum and thigh is inspected for any lesions. Inguinal glands are palpated and pubic hair is examined for lice. The labia minora are then separated and the urethral meatus is wiped clean. The meatus and para-urethral ducts (Skene's glands) are visualised and inspected. The labia majora is palpated and the condition of the Bartholin's glands noted. Tenderness is indicative of current infection and the glands may be swollen.

A speculum is then inserted into the vagina and the surface characteristics of the vagina and cervix are inspected. The cervix usually looks pink, feels firm and mobile without lesions; it may be round or slit-shaped. The vaginal surface is rugous (ridged) and moist. Any discharge should be sampled for culture and smear. The procedure for passing a speculum and obtaining vaginal, cervical and urethral specimens differs slightly from clinic to clinic. The procedure for testing the vaginal pH and the sniff, whiff or amine test can be found

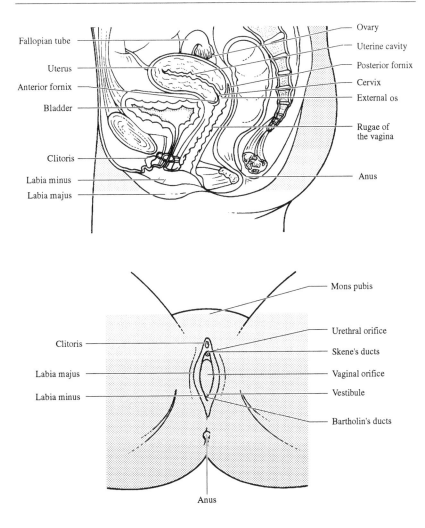

Fallopian tube
Uterus
Anterior fornix
Bladder
Clitoris
Labia minus
Labia majus

Ovary
Uterine cavity
Posterior fornix
Cervix
External os
Rugae of
the vagina
Anus

Mons pubis

Clitoris
Labia majus
Labia minus

Urethral orifice
Skene's ducts
Vaginal orifice
Vestibule
Bartholin's ducts

Anus

Figure 1.6: Anatomy of the female genito-urinary tract

in the section on bacterial vaginosis in Chapter 7.

Bi-manual palpation may then be performed to assess the condition of the fallopian tubes and ovaries. Findings may denote past or present infection. Rectal examination may be performed to assess anal sphincter tone and surface characteristics. A rectal slide and swab may be requested if anal intercourse has taken place. A throat swab may be taken if oral sex (fellatio) has occurred. Finally, a general physical examination of other systems may be performed, looking especially for any signs of syphilis.

Male examination

Physical assessment of the male reproductive system begins with the inspection of the genital and inguinal area (see Figure 1.7 for the anatomy of the male genito-urinary tract). The doctor may wish to examine the male patient standing up or lying down. Lower garments need to be lowered or removed to expose the genital region for examination. On examination, the skin on and around the genitalia is inspected for any abnormalities, for example redness, scars, lesions, ulcers or breaks of any kind in the skin. The groins are then palpated for the lymph glands and the hair on the pubis and lower abdomen is examined for lice.

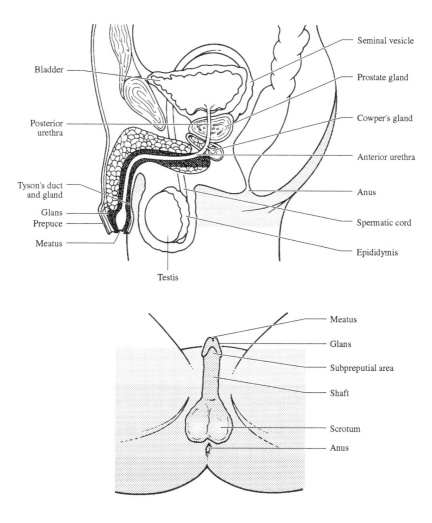

Figure 1.7: Anatomy of the male genito-urinary tract

In the uncircumcised male the prepuce is retracted and the condition of the prepuce, glans penis and the urethral meatus is noted. Characteristics of any urethral discharge, if present, are documented. Inability to retract the prepuce from the glans occurs sometimes in the uncircumcised man. This may cause a build-up of secretions (smegma) and may lead to inflammation of the tissues. Inability of the retracted prepuce to return to its normal position over the glans penis (paraphimosis) could, if untreated, impair local circulation, lead to oedema and even gangrene of the glans penis. Genital specimens are obtained from the urethral meatus and are sent for microscopy and culture.

Other areas of the body may be tested, depending on the nature of sexual activity, for example a subpreputial, rectal or throat swab may be taken. Prostatic massage may also be required. A gloved, lubricated index finger is inserted into the rectum. Using the pad of the index finger the prostate gland is located and massaged gently (Morton, 1990). A specimen of prostatic fluid is then obtained from the urethral meatus and sent for microscopy and culture.

Other investigations

Depending on the patient's signs and symptoms, other investigations may be required instead of or alongside the routine STD screen. Anyone who has an ulceration of any degree may be required to undergo tests to exclude syphilis and herpes. X-rays and ultrasound scans may be requested and lumbar punctures, colposcopies and biopsies are not uncommon procedures in GUM.

Referrals to other specialities may be necessary, for example urology, obstetrics and gynaecology, family planning, dermatology, rheumatology, medicine and general surgery.

Microscopy

It is important to have Gram staining facilities in the GUM department so that prompt diagnosis and treatment can be offered. When the specimens have been obtained, the slides are stained, as shown in Figure 1.8 and an immediate presumptive diagnosis of gonococcal or non-gonococcal urethritis can be made. Candida and bacterial vaginosis can also be diagnosed in this way.

Phase contrast or dark-field microscopy is used to visualise treponemes and *Trichomonas vaginalis* on a wet mount. Again concurrent infection with candida and bacterial vaginosis may also be seen.

SPECIALIST CLINICAL PRACTICE

GRAM STAINING

Practice statement
To prepare and stain the slides correctly for oil immersion microscopy

Equipment
Non-sterile gloves
Slide tray
Bunsen burner (if available)
Staining rack
Running water
Blotting paper
Staining bottles containing:
    methyl violet/crystal violet
    Lugol's iodine
    acetone/95% ethanol
    neutral red/dilute carbol fuchsin

Action	Rationale
1 Air dry the slide thoroughly or heat gently by passing through a Bunsen burner flame	To fix the specimen on to the slide
2 Place the slide on the staining rack. Apply methyl violet. Leave for 1 minute	Stains all the organisms and the background purple
3 Wash off the methyl violet with water. Apply Lugol's iodine and leave it on for 2 minutes	Iodine fixes the methyl violet into the Gram-positive organisms
4 Wash the iodine off with acetone until no more colour comes away (approx. 2–3 secs). Put the slide under running water *immediately*	Acetone decolourises all the methyl violet from the background and Gram-negative organisms. Water stops the decolourisation process
5 Apply neutral red as a counter stain. Leave for 2 minutes	Stains the background and Gram-negative organisms red
6 Wash the neutral red off with water	To remove excess stain
7 Dry the slide by removing excess water with blotting paper	The slide needs to be dry ready for oil immersion microscopy

Note
'Gram-positive organisms stain blue or purple or black. Gram-negative organisms stain pink or red.' (Shanson, 1982)

Reference
Shanson DC (1985) Microbiology in Clinical Practice. Bristol: Wright.

Bibliography *(for clinical practice relating to Gram staining)*
Cruikshank R, Duguid JP, Marmion BP, Swain RHA (1973) Medical Microbiology. Edinburgh: Churchill Livingstone.
Finegold SM, Baron EJ (1986) Bailey and Scott's Diagnostic Microbiology, 7th edn. Missouri: The CV Mosby Co.

Figure 1.8: Specialist clinical practice for Gram staining

All diagnoses must be confirmed by culture or serological tests carried out by the appropriate laboratories (Schofield, 1979). Specimens may be plated on to selective media, for example Thayer-Martin, as soon as they are obtained or put into a transport media, for example Amies charcoal, where the organisms can survive for up to 24 hours before being plated.

Urinalysis

The urine is tested as part of the routine STD screening procedure and when carrying out tests of cure on men. Patients are advised to try not to pass urine for one to four hours prior to their appointment, so that any discharge will collect in the urethra. The urine is then tested after urethral specimens have been obtained. A two-glass urine test helps distinguish between anterior and posterior urethritis in a male patient (see Figure 1.9 for an example of this procedure from the authors' clinic).

Urine testing using multi-reagent strips is a routine procedure in all fields of nursing. However, its importance should not be under-estimated. When used correctly, reagent strips can provide a comprehensive urine screen much easier, quicker and cheaper than laboratory tests (Thompson, 1991). Research has shown that the presence of blood and protein in the urine may indicate a urinary tract infection. Sugar and ketones may be detected in the urine of someone with undiagnosed diabetes when they present at a GUM clinic with recurrent candida problems. For reagent strip tests to be accurate they must be stored correctly, used in accordance with the manufacturer's instructions and time intervals specified for the readings must be scrupulously observed (Cook, 1995).

If a specimen of urine is obviously infected or bloodstained, it should be sent to the laboratory for culture and sensitivity (Thompson, 1991). When a patient complains of dysuria or frequency of micturition a midstream specimen of urine (MSU) is obtained. Figure 1.10 shows this procedure from the authors' clinic.

A specimen of urine is often collected for pregnancy testing in the GUM clinic. Human chorionic gonadotrophin (hCG) is present in the urine of pregnant women and the latest pregnancy testing kits are very sensitive in detecting its presence, thus detecting pregnancy early. The package insert in the pack of hCG-urine tests will give detailed instructions on how to carry out the test and these must be followed precisely for an accurate result.

**THE ROYAL WOLVERHAMPTON HOSPITALS NHS TRUST
MEDICAL SPECIALIST CLINICAL PRACTICES
SUB COMMITTEE GROUP**

G U M Clinical Practices No. **3**
Ratified: **19.01.95**

TWO-GLASS URINE TEST

Practice statement

Obtaining a specimen of urine from male patients to differentiate between anterior urethritis and an upper urinary tract infection

Equipment

Non-sterile gloves
2 x clean urine glasses
Acetic acid 33%
Urine test strips (BM-Test-5L)

Note

The patient should be advised to hold his urine for at least 4 hours before attending the clinic, otherwise the test could be inaccurate. This allows for any discharge to collect within the urethra

Action	Rationale
1 Ask the patient to pass 2–3 inches (60–120 ml) of urine into the first glass, and the remainder of his specimen into the second glass	To obtain a sample of urine for testing
2 First glass	
a) Gently rotate the glass and observe the urine for threads or specks of pus. If there are some present, observe whether they float or sink to the bottom of the glass	The presence of threads and a hazy appearance in the first glass confirms urethritis
b) Observe the urine for cloudiness, and if it is so, add a few drops of acetic acid 33%. Note whether the cloudiness remains	If the urine clears with the addition of the acetic acid, then the cloudiness is due to the presence of phosphates – a normal phenomenon
3 Second glass	
a) Briefly (no longer than 1 second) dip the test strip into the urine. Wipe off the excess urine on the rim of the glass. After 60 seconds, compare the reaction colours with the colour scales on the label of the urine test strip bottle	To test the patient's urine for the presence of blood, protein, glucose and ketone bodies
b) Observe whether the urine is clear or cloudy, and whether it contains threads and other urinary debris	To confirm urethritis and exclude urinary tract infection

Figure 1.9: Specialist clinical practice for the two-glass urine test

4 Record your findings in the patient's notes	To provide a permanent record

Bibliography
(for clinical practice relating to two-glass urine test)
Adler MW (1990) ABC of Sexually Transmitted Diseases. 2nd edn. London: British Medical Association
Boehringer Manneheim UK (Diagnostics and Biochemicals) Ltd (1992) Information leaflet supplied with BM-Test-5L kit.
Newall RG, Howell R (1990) Clinical Urinalysis. Ames Division, Miles Limited
Schofield CBS (1979) Sexually Transmitted Diseases. 3rd edn. Edinburgh: Churchill Livingstone
Reproduced with the kind permission of The Royal Woverhampton Hospitals NHS Trust.

FOOTNOTE
This clinical practice is under review at the time of publishing. A recommendation is being made that uncircumcised patients retract the foreskin before passing urine.

Figure 1.9: *Continued* Reproduced with the kind permission of The Royal Wolverhampton Hospitals NHS Trust.

SPECIALIST CLINICAL PRACTICE

Collection of a clean midstream specimen of urine (MSU)
Practice statement
To collect a specimen of bladder urine uncontaminated by bacteria for microscopy examination

Equipment
'Uripot' midstream collection pack (containing aqueous towelette – benzyl alcohol)
or
Universal container
Sterile receiver
Cotton wool balls (moistened with warm water)
Cotton wool balls (moistened with antiseptic*) or soap

Action	**Rationale**
1 Assemble or prepare the equipment, taking care not to touch the inside of the receiver	To maintain asepsis
2 Ask the patient to wash their hands then: a) Instruct or assist the female patient to separate the labia minora with one hand. Using the other hand, cleanse the urethral meatus and	To remove bacteria from the skin and external genitalia

Figure 1.10: Specialist clinical practice for collecting a midstream specimen of urine

vestibule with the antiseptic/aqueous towelette by wiping towards the rectum with one stroke over the inner surface of the labia minora and over the urethral meatus. Repeat with cotton wool balls moistened with warm water

b) Instruct or assist the male patient to use one hand to retract the prepuce and expose the urethral meatus. (The prepuce is repositioned following specimen collection.) Using the other hand, cleanse the urethral meatus and glans with the antiseptic/aqueous towelette, starting at the meatus and going downwards in a circular motion. Repeat with cotton wool balls moistened with warm water — To rinse off the soap or antiseptic solution

3 The first 20 ml or so of the urine voided is not for MSU collection. The second specimen is collected in a sterile container. The remaining urine is voided in the lavatory. (If the specimen is collected in a sterile receiver, transfer urine into a sterile universal container) — To collect a midstream specimen of urine

4 Close the specimen container, taking care not to touch the inner surface of the lid — To avoid contamination of the specimen

5 Label the container and seal it in the microbiology bag attached to the completed form — To transport the specimen correctly and safely

6 Send the specimen to the laboratory for culturing within 1–2 hours of collection. Alternatively, refrigerate the specimen at 4–8 °C or preserve the specimen in boric acid prior to examination — To avoid contamination and ensure prompt culturing

* Note – Antiseptic solutions: Povidone iodine, Benzalkonium chloride, Hexachlorophine

An MSU from the male should be collected before prostatic examination to prevent contamination by prostatic secretions.

Bibliography
(relating to clinical practice for collection of a midstream specimen of urine)
Baerheim A (1992) Obtaining clean urine samples. Nursing Times 88(39): 55.
Karlowicz KA (1995) Urological Nursing; Principles and Practice. London: W B Saunders.
Siroky MB, Krane RJ (1990) Manual of Urology. London: Little Brown & Co.

Figure 1.10: *Continued* Reproduced with the kind permission of The Royal Wolverhampton Hospitals NHS Trust.

Venepuncture

Finally, to complete routine STD screening, a sample of blood is obtained from the patient in order to exclude syphilis. This procedure is referred to as a serological test for syphilis (STS). When *Treponema pallidum* invades human tissue, a complex antibody response takes place and the various serological tests detect one or more of these antibodies. When results are negative, it is sometimes recommended that a further blood sample is taken 3 months later, for confirmation.

Nurses who are responsible for performing venepuncture must ensure a safe and correct practice, an example of which is shown in Figure 1.11. Taking blood with vacuumed containers is now a widespread practice and this has minimised the risk of coming into direct contact with blood.

WOLVERHAMPTON ACUTE HOSPITALS
GENERAL CLINICAL PRACTICES
SUB COMMITTEE GROUP

Clinical Practice No **V/CP1**
Ratified: **10.02.94**

VENEPUNCTURE SARSTEDT SAFETY MONOVETTE

Practice statement
To ensure safe and correct venous blood collection for laboratory examination.

Equipment
Tourniquet
21G Needle
Appropriate syringe
Alcohol swab
Filmated swab
Small adhesive dressing
Pathology requisition form
Biohazard bag (if there is not one already attached to the form)

Action	Rationale
1 Apply tourniquet to the limb above site selected	To dilate the veins by obstructing venous return
2 Ask the patient to assist in dilating of veins by clenching and unclenching the fist	To increase the prominence of the veins
3 Select the vein to be used by palpating. The veins may be tapped lightly	To choose best vein, promote blood flow and therefore distend the veins

---

Figure 1.11: Clinical practice for venepuncture

4 Swab vein with alcohol swab and allow to dry	To clean the puncture site
5 a) If using monovette as a syringe: attach needle to syringe and remove needle guard.	To prepare equipment for use
b) If using monovette as a vacutainer: lock piston off syringe and break off plunger	To prepare equipment by obtaining a vacuum in syringe cavity
6 Slide the bevelled side of needle into the selected vein at an angle of approximately 30 degrees. Using the thumb of opposite hand pull skin forward and stabilise chosen vein	To ensure a successful, pain free venepuncture entry
7 a) If using monovette as a syringe: pull piston back and withdraw required volume of blood	To ensure correct amount of blood is obtained
b) If using monovette as a vacutainer: attach vacuumed syringe to needle and lock together	To ensure correct amount of blood is obtained
8 Release tourniquet and unlock syringe from needle	To decrease pressure in the vein, and to prevent blood escape on withdrawal
9 Place a swab over needle site and remove needle gently from vein, applying slight pressure on the swab	To prevent blood leakage and haematoma formation
10 If using as a syringe, click back monovette piston and break off plunger	To obtain a vacuum in syringe
11 Label syringe and pack appropriately for transportation to laboratory	To ensure blood is safely and correctly presented to laboratory
12 Inspect puncture site before applying a small adhesive dressing	To check bleeding has ceased at puncture site and prevent contamination

Note

In most circumstances the antecubital veins are the veins of choice, because of their wide lumens, thick walls and because the skin is less sensitive

Bibliography

(for clinical practice relating to venepuncture)

Humphries PJ (1990) Safe Blood Collection. London: Clinical Laboratory Practice.

Rowlands R (1991) Making sense of venepuncture. Nursing Times 87(32).

Sarstedt Safety Monovette Intructions for Use.

Thorpe S (1991) A Practical Guide to Taking Blood. London: Baillière Tindall.

Figure 1.11: *Continued* Reproduced with the kind permission of The Royal Wolverhampton Hospitals NHS Trust.

Blood samples other than for the STS may need to be taken, depending on the patient's symptoms, for example viral antibodies and full blood count. Following the patient's request and pre-test counselling, blood may also be sent for HIV antibody testing.

Treatment and follow-up

The GUM department usually stocks a range of antibiotics, antifungal agents and topical treatments to be given out as prescribed. All treatment is free of prescription charges. The nurse administering the medication must ensure that the patient knows when to take it or how to use it. Relevant information and advice is given regarding administration and possible side effects. Patients are advised to refrain from sexual intercourse until the course of treatment is complete and follow-up tests prove clear. Patients may be referred to the health adviser for contact tracing and any further information they might require. It is important that sexual contacts are advised to attend a clinic to control the spread of infection. Education is also an important control measure. Patients must be advised that the use of a barrier contraceptive, i.e. a condom, will reduce the risk of certain diseases (Adler, 1990).

A follow-up appointment is made to review the patient's condition, give results and perform tests of cure as necessary. It is important to ensure that the appointment time given is convenient for the patient and that he or she understands that the return visit should not take as long as the initial one.

References

Adimora AA, Hamilton H, Holmes KK, Sparling PF (1994) Sexually Transmitted Diseases: Companion Handbook, 2nd edn. New York: McGraw-Hill.
Adler MW (1990) ABC of Sexually Transmitted Diseases, 2nd edn. London: British Medical Association.
Allen I, Hogg D (1993) Work Roles and Responsibilities in Genitourinary Medicine Clinics. London: Policy Studies Institute.
Andrews S (1994) Nurse prescribing. In Hunt G, Wainwright P (Eds), Expanding the Role of the Nurse. Oxford: Blackwell Science.
Arya OP, Osoba AO, Bennett FJ (1988) Tropical Venereology. Edinburgh: Churchill Livingstone.
British Medical Association, General Medical Services Committee, Health Education Authority, Brook Advisory Centres, Family Planning Association, Royal College of General Practitioners (undated) Confidentiality and People Under 16. London: British Medical Association.
Castledine G (1994) Specialist and advanced nursing and the scope of practice. In Hunt G, Wainwright P (Eds), Expanding the Role of the Nurse. Oxford: Blackwell Science.

Cook R (1995) Urinalysis. Nursing Standard 9(28): 32–5.

DHSS (1989) The Extending Role of the Nurse. London: HMSO.

DOH (1988) Report of the Working Group to Examine Workloads in Genitourinary Medicine Clinics (The Monks Report). London: HMSO.

DOH (1992) The Patient's Charter: Raising the Standard. London: HMSO.

DOH (1993a) The Health of the Nation: Key Area Handbook HIV/AIDS and Sexual Health. London: HMSO.

DOH (1993b) A Vision for the Future. London: HMSO.

Friend B (1992) Record recovery. Nursing Times 88(2): 34–5.

Genito-Urinary Nurses Association (1995) Guidelines for Good Practice. GUNA.

Heywood Jones I (1989) Buried under paper. Nursing Times 85(34): 57–8.

Hulme N, Smith S, Barton SE (1992) Insurance and HIV antibody testing. Lancet 339: 682–3.

James T, Harding I, Corbett K (1994) Biased care? Nursing Times 90 (51): 28–31.

Kinnell H (1993) Wolverhampton Sex Workers Survey Report. Safe HIV Outreach Project, South Birmingham Health Authority.

Morton PG (1990) Health Assessment. Springhouse: Springhouse Corporation.

Palmer H (1995) Clinical supervision for nurses working with people with HIV/AIDS. Professional Nurse 11(1): 20–2.

Rogers JS, Adler MW (1987) Role and training of nurses working in departments of genitourinary medicine in England and Wales. Genitourinary Medicine 63: 122–32.

Schofield CBS (1979) Sexually Transmitted Diseases, 3rd edn. Edinburgh: Churchill Livingstone.

Thompson J (1991) The significance of urine testing. Nursing Standard 5(25): 39–40.

UKCC (1992a) Code of Professional Conduct, 3rd edn. London: UKCC.

UKCC (1992b) The Scope of Professional Practice. London: UKCC.

UKCC (1993) Standards for Records and Record Keeping. London: UKCC.

Additional reading

English National Board (1994) Caring for People with Sexually Transmitted Diseases, Including HIV Disease. Open learning pack. London: ENB.

Guilleband J (1993) Contraception – Your Questions Answered, 2nd edn. Edinburgh: Churchill Livingstone.

Health Education Council (1980) Handbook on Contact Tracing in Sexually Transmitted Diseases. London: HEC.

Hunt G, Wainwright P (1994) Expanding the Role of the Nurse. Oxford: Blackwell Science.

Useful addresses

English National Board for Nursing
Victory House, 170 Tottenham Court Road, London W1P 0HA

The Family Planning Association
27–35 Mortimer Street, London W1N 7RJ

Genito-urinary Nurses Association (GUNA)
For details contact GUNA membership secretary: Mrs Gay Lacy, Sister,
Department of Genito-Urinary Medicine, Taunton & Somerset Hospital,
Musgrove Park, Taunton TA1 5DA

The Health Education Authority
Hamilton House, Mabledon Place, London WC1H 9TX

Royal College of Nursing
20 Cavendish Square, London W1M 9AE

United Kingdom Central Council for Nursing, Midwifery and Health Visiting
23 Portland Place, London W1N 3AF

Appendix: Specialist clinical practices for the collection of specimens

THE ROYAL WOLVERHAMPTON HOSPITALS
NHS TRUST
MEDICAL SPECIALIST CLINICAL PRACTICES
SUB COMMITTEE GROUP

G U M Clinical Practices No. **5**
Ratified: **19.01.95**

Information package and practice relating to collection of specimens in the Department of Genito-Urinary Medicine

Practice statement
To obtain uncontaminated specimens, as requested by the doctor (to aid/confirm
diagnosis) with minimal discomfort to the patient

IMPORTANT INFORMATION

Labelling specimens
Before taking any specimens, ensure that all slides and culture bottles are clearly
marked with the patient's GUM Clinic number. In order to maintain confidential-
ity, patient's names are never used
Microscopy slides are labelled using a chinagraph pencil
Culture transport media bottles are labelled with printed labels

Control of infection
If there is any clinical suspicion that a patient is infected with hepatitis B virus or
human immunodeficiency virus (HIV) the staff must adhere to the Control of
Infection Policy No 21 (Policy for the hospital care of patients infected with or
carriers of hepatitis B virus or HIV)

Please note
When performing urethral tests, urine should not be passed for 2–3 hours prior to
obtaining a swab in order to avoid organisms being flushed away

MALE TESTS

Obtaining urethral specimens

Equipment
Non-sterile latex gloves
2 Microscopy slides
1 Cover slip
*1 Sterile wire swab and tube containing Amies charcoal transport medium
1 Bottle of chlamydia culture transport medium
**1 Sterile wire swab
Normal saline
Scissors
Anglepoise lamp

Action	Rationale
1 If the patient has not been circumcised, ask him to retract the foreskin	To expose the urethra
2 Ask the patient to gently part the meatus	To ensure maximum visibility of the area to be swabbed
3 **a**) Insert a sterile swab* into the meatus, approximately 1.5–2 cm deep, and rotate it gently	To obtain the required specimen and prepare it for microscopy and culture
b) Spread some of the sample obtained out thinly on to a dry glass slide, then dip the swab on to the wet glass slide (moistened with a drop of normal saline) and apply the cover slip. Insert the swab into the Amies charcoal trans port medium	

To obtain a specimen for chlamydia:

4 Insert sterile wire swab** into the meatus, approximately 2 cm deep, and rotate it twice. Withdraw the swab and place it directly in to the chlamydia culture transport medium	To obtain the required specimen for chlamydia culture

Note
If a specimen is required for 'immunofluorescence', then some of the sample must be spread on to the immunofluorescence slide before inserting the swab into the transport medium

FOOTNOTE
This clinical practice is under review at the time of publishing. It is being recommended that plastic loops are used to obtain specimens for microscopy rather than wire swabs

Obtaining a subpreputial specimen

Equipment
Non-sterile latex gloves
1 Microscopy slide
1 Sterile wire swab and tube containing Amies charcoal transport medium

Action	**Rationale**
1 If the patient has not been circumcised, ask him to retract the foreskin	To ensure maximum visibility of the area to be sampled
2 Scrape a sterile swab gently over the preputial sac	To obtain the required specimen
3 Spread some of the sample obtained out thinly on to a dry glass slide, and then insert the swab directly in to the Amies charcoal transport medium	To prepare the specimen for microscopy and culture

Notes
1. If the preputial sac is dry, the swab could be moistened in normal saline prior to taking the specimen.
2. A wet film could be taken from the subpreputial sac, if required by the doctor. (Refer to 'Obtaining urethral specimens' **3b**)

FEMALE TESTS

Obtaining vaginal, cervical and urethral specimens

Equipment
Non-sterile latex gloves
3 Plain microscopy slides
1 Chlamydia slide
1 Cover slip
2 Sterile paper swabs with tubes of Amies charcoal medium
1 Sterile wire swab with tube of Amies charcoal medium
1 Single paper swab
1 Bottle of chlamydia culture transport medium

Normal saline
Bi-valve speculae
Sponge-holding forceps
Non-sterile cotton wool balls
Lubricating jelly (optional)
Receiver
Adjustable light

Action	Rationale
1 Assist the patient into the lithotomy position. Wipe away any secretions from the vulval area using a downward movement from the clitoris to the perineum	To enable inspection of the genital area and remove any excess secretions
2 Insert the speculae gently into the vaginal orifice. When fully inserted, open the speculae and locate the cervix. When the cervix is positioned between the open blades, tighten the screw on the speculae to fix it in position	To ensure maximum visibility of the area to be inspected and swabbed

Vaginal slides and swabs

3 a) Take two glass slides – leave one dry, and apply 1 drop of normal saline to make the other one wet	To obtain specimens from the vagina and prepare them ready for microscopy and culture
b) Using a paper swab, swab the lateral vaginal walls and spread the specimen evenly on to the dry glass slide	
c) Using the same swab, swab the posterior fornix; then dip it into the solution on the wet slide and apply a cover slip. Next, place the swab directly into Amies charcoal medium	

Cervical slides and swabs

4 a) If necessary, gently clean the cervix using the sponge-holding forceps and a cotton wool ball	To ensure maximum visibility of the cervical os
b) Insert a sterile paper swab into the cervical os, and rotate it twice	To obtain an adequate specimen
c) Spread some of the sample obtained on to the glass slide, and then place the swab directly into the Amies charcoal medium	To prepare the specimen for testing
d) Repeat 4b with another paper swab. Rotate swab twice against the endo cervix. Then place the swab into the chlamydia culture transport medium	To obtain an optimum amount of endocervical cells for chlamydia culture

Urethral slides and swabs

5 a) Insert a sterile wire swab into the urethra for 1 cm in an upward and backward direction, and rotate the swab very gently	To obtain the required specimen
b) Spread the specimen evenly on to the chlamydia and microscopy slides and then place it directly into the Amies charcoal medium	To prepare the specimen for chlamydia immunofluorescence, microscopy and culture

MALE/FEMALE TESTS

Obtaining a rectal slide and swab

Equipment
Non-sterile latex gloves
Lubricating jelly
Disposable proctoscope
Light source/adjustable light
1 Microscopy slide
1 Sterile swab and Amies charcoal transport medium
Tissues

Action	Rationale
1 a) **(Male)** Assist the patient into the left lateral position and ask him to draw his knees up to his abdomen b) **(Female)** A woman may be examined in the lithotomy position if she finds it more comfortable	To ensure maximum visibility of the area to be examined and to ensure maximum safety for the patient during the procedure
2 Lubricate the proctoscope and insert it gently into the anus, and ask the patient to bear down. When the proctoscope is fully inserted, remove the introducer and attach the light source (if available)	In order to relax the anal sphincter and be able to examine the appearance of the rectal mucosa
3 Using a sterile swab, swab the rectum with care. Then, withdraw the swab and remove the proctoscope gently, inspecting the rectal mucosa as you do so	To obtain the required sample and to visualise the rectal mucosa
4 Spread the sample obtained onto a glass slide and then put the swab directly into the Amies charcoal medium	To prepare the specimens for testing
5 Wipe away any excess lubricant around the anus	To make the patient comfortable

Note
At the discretion of the examiner, a blind swab (without using a proctoscope) may be taken

FOOTNOTE
In patients suspected of having thread worms, stick a piece of sellotape onto the perianal region, peel it off and then stick it onto a slide for microscopic examination

Obtaining a throat swab

Equipment
Non-sterile latex gloves
Tongue depressor
Sterile swab
Appropriate transport medium
Light source

Action	**Rationale**
1 Ask the patient to sit with the head bent slightly backwards, facing a strong light source. Ask the patient to open his/her mouth wide	To ensure maximum visibility of the throat
2 Depress the tongue slightly with the tongue depressor, and then quickly, but gently, rub the swab over the prescribed area (usually the tonsils) or any area with a lesion or visible exudate. See diagram below	To obtain the required sample
3 When collecting the specimen, avoid touching any other area of the mouth or tongue with the swab. Insert the swab immediately into the culture transport medium	To prevent contamination by other organisms

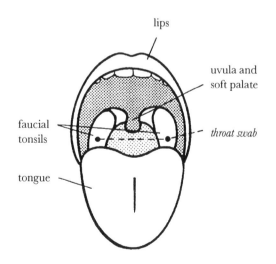

lips

uvula and
soft palate

faucial
tonsils

throat swab

tongue

Obtaining a specimen of serum for dark-field investigation

Equipment
Non-sterile latex gloves
2 Microscopy slides
2 Cover slips
Sachet of normal saline
Sterile gauze swabs
Sterile gallipot
Adjustable light

Action	Rationale
1 Swab the lesion with normal saline	To remove the surface debris
2 Put a drop of normal saline on each slide	To assist in microscopy
3 Gently squeeze the base of the lesion to ooze serum, and using a plastic loop collect a drop of serum and mix with the drop of saline. Alternatively, using a cover slip, scrape the exudate from the top of the lesion and smear it onto the glass slide into the saline. Place the cover slip on top	To obtain a suitable sample of material for microscopy
4 Repeat step 3	To confirm the examination result
5 Explain to the patient that this test may need to be repeated on 3 consecutive days	To confirm or exclude the diagnosis

Obtaining a specimen of serum for a Diff-Quick test

Equipment
Non-sterile gloves
1 Microscopy slide (preferably a chlamydia slide)
1 Cover slip
Sterile gallipot
Sterile gauze swabs
Sachet of normal saline
Adjustable light

Action	Rationale
1 Cleanse the lesion with swabs of gauze soaked in normal saline, then gently pat it dry	To remove the surface debris
2 Gently scrape the edge of the cover slip over the top of the lesion and smear the cells on to a dry slide. Allow to air dry	To obtain a sample of material for microscopy
3 Dispose of the cover slip in the sharps box	To prevent cross-infection and maintain staff safety

Obtaining a specimen for viral culture

Equipment
Non-sterile latex gloves
Sterile swab
Viral culture transport medium
Scissors
Adjustable light

Action	Rationale
1 Firmly swab the lesion, taking care not to touch the surrounding skin. Place the swab directly into the transport medium, and cut the stem short enough to fit inside the bottle	To obtain an uncontaminated specimen for culture
2 Store the specimen in the refrigerator until it is sent to the laboratory	To prolong viral survival

Despatch of specimens to the laboratory

Practice statement
To ensure that all specimens are transported safely to the appropriate laboratory

Equipment
Boxes for transporting slides
Biohazard bags
Request forms (with bag attached)
Biohazard labels
Metal transport tin

Action	Rationale
1 Ensure that all specimens are labelled correctly and that request forms are complete and correspond with the specimens and bear the doctor's signature	To avoid errors being made
2 Identify any patients who are: - HIV antibody positive - hepatitis B antigen positive - partners of the above - people who have been exposed to high risk activity in connection with HIV/hepatitis B Ensure that all their specimens and request forms are marked 'BIOHAZARD'	To ensure awareness of biohazard nature and protection to those who handle the specimens, should leakage of a specimen occur
3 Check that the tops on the culture bottles/tubes are secure before putting the specimens into sealed biohazard bags with the request forms attached. Slides	To prevent the specimens from leaking, and to maintain staff safety

should be slotted into the appropriate
boxes for transport, with the tops secured

4   All specimens are then to be put into the   To ensure safe transportation of
    appropriate sealed metal box for trans-   the specimens
    portation to the laboratory by the Hotel
    Services Department

Bibliography and suggested reading

(for clinical practices relating to the collection of specimens)

Adimora AA, Hamilton H, Holmes KK, Sparling PF (1994) Sexually Transmitted
    Diseases Companion Handbook. New York: McGraw-Hill.
Adler MW (1990) ABC of Sexually Transmitted Diseases, 2nd edn. London:
    British Medical Association.
Booth JA (1983) Handbook of Investigations. London: Harper & Row Limited.
Brunner LS, Suddarth DS (1982) The Lippincott Manual of Nursing Practice, 3rd
    edn. Philadelphia: JB Lippincott Company.
Chilman AM, Thomas M (1981) Understanding Nursing Care, 2nd edn.
    Edinburgh: Churchill Livingstone.
Jamieson EM, McCall JM, Blythe R, Logan WW (1988) Guide-lines for Clinical
    Nursing Practices. Edinburgh: Churchill Livingstone.
Pritchard AP, David JA (1988) The Royal Marsden Hospital Manual of Clinical
    Nursing Procedures, 2nd edn. London: Harper & Row Publishers.
Rambo BJ (1985) Nursing Skills for Clinical Practice, vol 3. Philadelphia: WB
    Saunders Company.
Schofield CBS (1979) Sexually Transmitted Diseases, 3rd edn. Edinburgh:
    Churchill Livingstone.
Stilwell B (1992) Skills Update. London: Macmillan Magazines Limited.
Wolverhampton Health Authority (1990) Control of Infection Policies 4, 12 & 21.

Reproduced with the kind permission of The Royal Woverhampton Hospitals
NHS Trust.

Chapter 2
Cytology and colposcopy

Sally-Ann Palmer

Cytology

Introduction

Cancer of the cervix has been an important issue in women's health for most of the twentieth century. The disease often used to go undetected until identifiable symptoms had appeared. As a result the disease was too far advanced for treatments to be effective, leading to a high mortality rate. Twenty per cent of all cancer in women is from cancer of the cervix and the uterus (Hope-Stone, 1990).

Chomet and Chomet (1991) noted that there were nearly half a million new cases of cervical cancer worldwide and that 60–90% of the women who died from cervical cancer had never had a smear. Hope-Stone (1990) notes that 95% of cases of cancer of the cervix occur in women over 30 years old, although carcinoma in situ, cervical intraepithelial neoplasia (CIN) and invasive cancer may occur in women under 35 years old.

Papanicolaou and Traut (1941) believed that the collection and examination of vaginal smears would allow treatment of cervical cancer to be given in the early pre-invasive stage, thus preventing the onset of carcinoma of the cervix. They felt that this would have a direct effect on reducing the incidence of mortality from the disease. Many years later their advice was followed with the development of national screening programmes.

Cervical cancer is normally either squamous carcinoma originating from the squamous epithelium or adenocarcinoma from the columnar epithelium. Peel (1995) notes that around 10% of cervical cancer is adenocarcinoma but that the percentage is rising. It has long been thought that cervical cancer starts as pre-cancer and that such pre-cancerous cells show that they might become cancerous by the uncontrolled multiplying of their cells. The cancerous masses that are formed can grow into the cervix and then beyond it into other organs, and cancerous cells may spread to other parts of the body through the lymphatic system causing metastases.

The female genital tract

Within the female genital tract there are three types of lining, each of which has a specific function. The squamous epithelium lines the vagina and part of the cervix in the vagina. It is a good protective layer and is able to withstand a lot of friction, such as that caused by intercourse. The endocervical epithelium lines the cervical canal. It is made up of columnar cells and contains glands that secrete mucus to lubricate the genital tract. It is much thinner and more friable than squamous epithelium. The uterus is lined by endometrium, which also contains a lot of glands. Chomet and Chomet (1991) note that the influence of ovarian and pituitary hormones which determine the thickness of the endometrium, the secretion of fluids and cell growth mean that the linings of the female genital tract are in a constant state of change.

Pre-cancerous changes mostly occur either at the point where the two different types of lining in the cervix meet, called the squamo-columnar junction (SCJ) or at the transformation zone. In childhood the SCJ is found in the cervical canal. During puberty and adolescence, under the influence of oestrogen, the SCJ moves down and out on to the vaginal surface of the cervix. This is known as ectopy. The columnar cells that are exposed are affected by the acidity of the vagina and the process of squamous metaplasia takes place, which changes columnar epithelium into squamous epithelium. The transformation zone is the area on the cervix between the site of the original squamous epithelium and original columnar epithelium (Evans, 1990). This process is reversed after the menopause, when the epithelium reduces in size and the SCJ and transformation zone move back into the cervical canal, often high up (Chomet & Chomet, 1991). Ulmer (1994) states that squamous metaplasia is a normal process that does not necessarily lead to the development of pre-cancer or cancer. Soutter (1993) observes that dysplasia in the form of CIN develops when metaplasia is disturbed in some way. Figure 2.1 shows the cervix and the transformation zone.

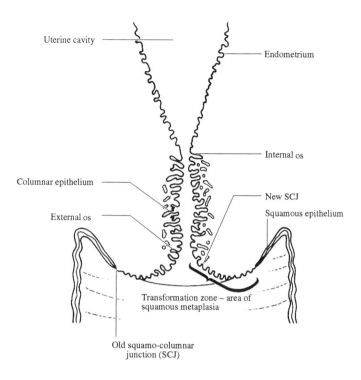

Figure 2.1: Cervix and transformation zone.

The cervical smear and screening

In the USA the examination of the cervix is often known as the Pap smear test or Pap test (Ulmer, 1994). However, in this country it is usually referred to as a cervical smear or cytology. The cervical smear involves scraping cells from the SCJ, smearing the cells on to a glass slide and then fixing the specimen with 95% ethyl alcohol or a similar fixative from an aerosol (Peel, 1995). The slide is then stained and examined under a microscope in a cytology laboratory for abnormal cells. Changes are graded according to the degree of severity, and it is important to remember that an abnormal smear only rarely means that actual cancer of the cervix is present.

There have been various initiatives recently to encourage the uptake of cervical screening in an attempt to reduce the number of deaths from cervical cancer. *The Health of the Nation* document (DOH, 1993) set a target of a 20% reduction in the incidence of cervical cancer, in women of all ages, by the year 2000 from a 1986 baseline. The development of good practice in operating the screening programme and encouraging women to be screened were set as priorities by the government. Chomet and Chomet (1991) note that the British Society of Clinical Cytology has produced a standard terminology for reporting smear results. Smears are reported as negative if they are normal or contain cells showing inflammatory changes while those smears showing cells with an abnormal nucleus or dyskaryosis are graded as mild, moderate or severe (Peel, 1995).

Pre-cancerous changes

The term pre-cancer is used to describe a number of abnormalities that occur in the cervical epithelium but which are still confined to the epithelium (Chomet & Chomet, 1991). The general term used to describe the full range of changes is cervical intraepithelial neoplasia or CIN. Most abnormal cervical smears show non-invasive, pre-cancerous lesions which are easy to treat if diagnosed early. Changes in the nuclei of cells, related to future pre-cancerous and cancerous conditions, are noted on cervical smears and the dyskaryotic changes are reported as mild, moderate or severe. Mild dyskaryosis can be reversible and does not always progress to cancer. Moderate or severe dyskaryosis is more likely to lead to cancerous changes. If pre-cancerous cells are removed or destroyed, regardless of the degree of dyskaryosis present, then progression to cancer will be stopped (Chomet & Chomet, 1991).

Other changes may also be seen, such as a koilocyte, which is a cell whose nucleus appears to be surrounded by a halo of cytoplasm. The human papilloma virus (HPV) has been shown to cause koilocyte change to cells, though it does not cause all such haloes (Husain, 1990). He also notes that there appears to be a faster growing form of cancer developing in young women.

Predisposing factors for cervical cancer

There are a number of factors that appear to predispose a woman to developing cervical cancer.

Sexual intercourse and age of first intercourse

It has been known since the last century that sexual intercourse is a factor in cervical cancer (Husain, 1990) and the age of first intercourse is an important part of it. Chomet and Chomet (1991) point out that the younger a woman starts to have sex, the more partners she is likely to have. Some authors believe that the immature genital tract is more susceptible to cervical cancer (Farlow, 1993), but Chomet and Chomet (1991), along with many other authors, believe that the number of sexual partners is a more important factor. Some researchers believe that the change in sexual conventions in young people in the UK in the 1960s is the main reason why women aged 20–30 have shown a 3–4 times higher incidence of pre-cancerous changes over the last 10–15 years (Husain, 1990). Chomet and Chomet (1991) also show that a woman is more at risk if her partner has had many partners.

Smoking

Barton et al. (1988) suggest that the end result of HPV infection may be influenced by other factors in the body, such as smoking. It appears that cervical cells extract substances such as tobacco toxins from the blood and because they are concentrated in the cervix this may exacerbate the effects of other factors (Chomet & Chomet, 1991). Barton et al. (1988) found that smokers have fewer Langerhans' cells in the cervical epithelium than non-smokers and this may explain why smoking is a factor in the development of CIN.

Pregnancy

Although it is not clear why pregnancy should be a risk factor, endo-cervical cells are more exposed during pregnancy, which might make the cervix more vulnerable to infection (Farlow, 1993). However, Chomet and Chomet (1991) note that researchers are divided on whether having a first pregnancy under the age of 20 or having a large number of pregnancies are risk factors.

Occupation and social class

There is clear evidence that social class has an effect on the prevalence of cervical cancer, and British mortality statistics show cervical cancer to have the steepest social class gradient of any cancer (Peel, 1995). Austoker (1994) quantifies the risk stating that women in social class V are three times more likely to have cervical cancer than women in social class I. However, women in the lower socio-economic groups are the least likely to have a cervical smear carried out. Cervical cancer has been linked to poverty and women in the lower social classes are often in poorer health with lowered immune resistance to disease. They often marry young, divorce more often and have partners working in heavy industry or working away from home (Farlow, 1993).

    Peel (1995) notes that exposure of the male partner to substances such as coal tar or mineral oil may be relevant. The heavy metal ions in such substances may be carcinogenic (Farlow, 1993). Chomet and Chomet (1991) also note that women who work in the textile industry are thought to be at higher risk of cervical cancer. It is believed this work exposes women to oil from textile wastes, which may be taken in through the skin and concentrated in the cervix or possibly transmitted to the genital area from the hands.

Genetic factors

Farlow (1993) suggests that histones or proteins found in the head of the sperm of some men prevent the DNA mechanism in cells of the cervix from functioning correctly. Peel (1995) notes that this factor might involve the male partner and the environment as well as the woman.

Viral factors

Peel (1995) notes that many women with asymptomatic CIN have evidence of HPV infection on cytology, colposcopy and in biopsy specimens. HPV types 6, 11, 16 and 18 have all been identified with genital warts, pre-cancer change and cervical cancer. The occurrence of sexually transmitted HPV infections has been reported to have increased. Between 1984 and 1994 the number of new cases seen in genito-urinary medicine (GUM) clinics nearly doubled to 86 725 in 1994 (DOH, 1995). Mela (1993) suggests that teenage patients of GPs should be educated about the risk of HPV and cervical cancer, just as they are educated about smoking.

High titres of antibodies to *Herpes simplex* virus (HSV) type II have been found in women with CIN or cervical cancer (Peel, 1995). However, he also notes that there are conflicting reports about the relevance of this and it may be that the antibody tests are not specific enough.

Contraception

Hare (1990) believes that there have not been any large-scale studies of the effectiveness of condoms in preventing sexually transmitted diseases (STDs), though small studies suggest that condoms definitely protect against STDs. Chomet and Chomet (1991) suggest that it is arguable whether the use of the contraceptive pill is linked to an increased risk of cervical cancer. However, if barrier methods of contraception are used then there is a lower incidence of cervical cancer, maybe because semen, bacteria and viruses are prevented from reaching the cervix.

Drugs

Many immunosuppressive drugs are now used in transplant surgery and in the medical treatment of auto-immune diseases, for example ulcerative colitis, thyroid disorders and rheumatoid arthritis (Chomet & Chomet, 1991). Because the immune system in women taking such drugs is altered, they could be at greater risk of developing cervical cancer. It is believed also that drugs such as heroin used by injecting drug users can have a detrimental effect on the immune system (Chomet & Chomet, 1991). Many GUM clinics see drug users as patients and nurses should be aware of this factor in cervical cancer.

Vitamin and mineral deficiencies

Held (1995) notes that the lack of certain vitamins and minerals including vitamins A, C, folic acid and selenium are thought to have a role in the development of cervical cancer.

Penile hygiene and cancer

A woman whose partner has poor penile hygiene or penile cancer or whose previous partner had cervical cancer appears to be at greater risk of developing cervical cancer (Chomet & Chomet, 1991; Held, 1995).

The recall system

The recall system is designed to allow cytology units in pathology departments to follow up patients with overdue smears, abnormal smears, those women who need repeat smears or who have had or need colposcopy undertaken. The system checks on smears taken in any venue, including GP surgeries, gynaecological (gynae) outpatients, family planning clinics, gynae wards, antenatal wards or GUM, within that particular health authority.

Confidentiality is of paramount importance for patients attending GUM clinics. However, it is important to inform GPs of smear results to ensure that patients, who may move around the country, are followed up and repeat smears or treatment are carried out if necessary. In GUM the patient must give permission before the GP is informed of her smear result. Confidentiality means that the GP is only given the smear or colposcopy result and not information about infections or other tests carried out, unless the patient requests this. It is important that GUM clinics are sensitive to the fact that GP practices are the main centres where smears are taken. A GUM clinic will normally take a smear at the request of a patient or if the doctor considers that it should be done as part of the GU screen. Some clinics routinely take a smear from a woman who has not had a smear taken before to ensure that the woman is then part of the recall system and is regularly reminded to have smears. Some GUM clinics record in a smear book the patient number, the date and the name of the person taking the smear for audit purposes and to ensure good practice in taking smears. When the smear result is sent to GUM, it is checked by a doctor or nurse, depending on the clinic policy and recorded in the notes. If a recall smear has been requested by the cytologists or colposcopy or other treatment is recommended, this information is recorded either on computer or in a book so that future follow-up is undertaken.

The screening programme

Peel (1995) states that to be considered effective, a screening programme should reduce both the incidence of cervical cancer and mortality from the disease. Screening programmes have been running for over 30 years in the USA and Canada and for 20 years in some European countries, including Britain. Cervical screening programmes in Iceland, Finland, Sweden and parts of Denmark, where there has been complete coverage of the target population, have led to a dramatic drop in both the incidence and the mortality (Austoker, 1994).

In the UK generally, excluding the north east of Scotland, screening has been considered fairly ineffective and a relative failure in comparison with other countries, due to the poor implementation of the programme (Peel, 1995). Austoker (1994) suggests that the problems with the UK system were due to lack of organisation, accountability and commitment. In 1988 a computerised call and recall system was introduced based on the registers of age and sex held by Family Practitioner Committees in each of the NHS districts (Husain, 1990; Austoker,1994). In 1990, the government set targets for payment for GPs for cervical screening, which mean that all women aged between 20 and 60 in Scotland and 20 and 64 in England on a GP's list must be offered screening and 80% of the target population must be screened in the preceding five and a half years for the GP to receive full payment (Milburn & MacAskill, 1994); 33% of the full payment is made if only 50% of the target population is screened.

Austoker (1994) notes that following the setting of these targets there has been a real increase in screening, with 83% of GPs reaching the 80% target in October 1993, as opposed to only 53% in April 1990, and only 3% of GPs failed to reach either 50% or 80% screening in 1993, compared with 15% in 1990.

Age and frequency of screening

It must be recognised that cost will have an influence on the recommended screening programme (Peel, 1995). Husain (1990) notes that generally, preinvasive lesions develop 3–5 years after sexual activity starts and therefore, given present sexual practices, women should be screened when they are 20 years old. The International Agency for Research on Cancer (IARC) working group evaluated 10 established screening programmes by using case control studies (IARC, 1986) and showed that for 3 years after a negative smear protection against cervical cancer is high but after that it falls with time. They concluded that if women aged 35–64 were screened every 5 years it would protect 84% of women from cervical cancer; 3-yearly smears would protect 91% of women; and annual smears would protect 93.5% of women. As Husain (1990) says, annual smears are too expensive, 5-yearly screening is not frequent enough and allows cancer to develop, therefore 3-yearly screening would seem to be a good compromise and should be aimed at women aged 35–60, though screening should start before the age of 35 (IARC, 1986). Most clinicians consider that women who have never had sexual intercourse are at low risk of cervical cancer, though adenocarcinoma may be found in women who are virgins (Chomet & Chomet, 1991).

Preparing to take a smear

Various information is needed to fill out a cytology form. The patient is asked for the date of the first day of her last menstrual period; what contraception she uses – particularly oral contraception and intrauterine devices (IUDs); if she is on hormonal treatment other than for contraception; the date of her last cervical smear – if she has not had a smear before then that will be put on the form; and if she has had any intermenstrual, post-coital or post-menopausal bleeding. Chomet and Chomet (1991) also suggest that a woman be asked about her own and her partner's occupations, the number of pregnancies including miscarriage and abortion she has had and about any gynaecological abnormalities. However, whether this information is requested will depend on the policy of each particular district and the forms that are used.

The slide must be prepared with the patient's name or clinic number according to clinic policy, date of birth and usually the date the test is carried out.

It is important that a woman does not have a smear taken during her menstrual period as the smear may be difficult to read because of red blood cells. The epithelial cells that are sampled in cytology may be replaced by endometrial cells from the uterus if a smear is taken too close to menstruation. Therefore mid-cycle is an ideal time for taking a smear.

Chomet and Chomet (1991) suggest that condoms should be used for a few days before a smear is taken so sperm are not seen on the smear. However, this is relatively difficult to achieve in GUM. Chomet and Chomet (1991) also note that contraceptive cream used with a diaphragm or cap can affect a smear. This is more likely to be a problem in family planning clinics than in GUM. Many GUM clinics do not take a smear on the first visit if a discharge is present but do one at a follow-up visit after treatment has been given.

There are also different opinions about oral contraceptives. Some clinics consider that if an abnormal smear has been reported, oral contraceptives can be continued as usual, even following treatment for CIN, unless there are other reasons unconnected with the CIN for it to be discontinued. Other clinics consider the oral contraceptive to be contraindicated when CIN is being treated and prefer to recommend barrier methods of contraception.

Preparing the patient

Having a cervical smear is a very personal experience and many women do not like having an internal examination. The procedure of inserting the speculum is not comfortable but it should not hurt. It is important to explain the procedure to the patient, not only to help make it a less unpleasant experience but also to get the patient's co-operation and to encourage her to be as relaxed as possible. Milburn and MacAskill (1994) note how important it is for women to understand that cytology is done to detect pre-cancer not cancer and that many women are unaware of this. Cytology should not be referred to as a cancer smear as this gives a negative message and leads to confusion. It is important to treat the whole woman and have regard for her feelings. The nurse should be sensitive to the patient's possible embarrassment and allow her privacy to get undressed, if at all possible, to put her at ease.

McKie (1993) found that 65% of the women sampled in her study wanted to have their smear taken by a woman rather than a man. It is important, therefore, to arrange facilities within the clinic to enable a woman to have a smear taken either by a female doctor or nurse.

Emptying the bladder prior to a smear being taken will make the examination more comfortable. However, if routine GUM screening is also being undertaken this may not be possible.

Taking a cervical smear

Many GUM clinics have couches that put the patient into a modified lithotomy position. If this is not available the patient needs to lie back on an examination couch with her knees bent and dropped well apart in a relaxed position. Table 2.1 lists the equipment needed for taking a cervical smear. A blanket or drawsheet may be placed across the patient's abdomen. The doctor or nurse normally inspects the genital area for warts, rashes, discharge or spots (Chomet & Chomet, 1991). When a smear is done by a doctor in GUM, the doctor may do a pelvic examination, normally after the smear has been taken or when all the routine GUM tests are finished. The index and middle fingers of one hand are carefully inserted into the vagina and the other hand is placed over the abdomen. The doctor is usually able to feel the size, shape and position of the uterus, tubes and ovaries and may be able to feel changes in the anatomy, such as uterine fibroids, thickening of the tubes and ovarian cysts. Chomet and Chomet (1991) feel that not performing an internal examination when a woman is attending for a smear may mean that abnormalities are missed. However, if a nurse is taking a smear in GUM it is unlikely that she will do an internal examination.

Once the external genitalia have been checked the labia are gently opened and a closed bi-valve speculum is inserted into the vagina and carefully opened to part the vaginal walls and allow the cervix to be visualised high up inside the vagina. The speculum should be the right size, using as small a speculum as possible. Ideally it should not be lubricated or it should be lubricated with the smallest amount of lubricant possible as if too much is used this can interfere with the sample. Some clinics that use metal speculae warm them so they are not too cold.

The cervix and vagina are then checked and the smear is taken using a spatula or cytobrush to make two 360 degree sweeps of the

Table 2.1: Equipment for taking a cervical smear

- gloves
- spatulas, cytobrushes
- speculae of various sizes, placed in a container of warm water if metal
- KY jelly for lubrication (optional)
- good light source
- sponge forceps
- cotton wool
- glass cytology slides
- marker pencil/pen and rubber
- cervical smear fixative
- cervical smear cytology form
- slide holder
- cervical smear test leaflet, according to local policy
- blanket/drawsheet, according to clinic policy

transformation zone and the surface of the SCJ, wherever it is situated on the cervix.

Husain (1990) states that the material from both sides of the spatula must be spread on to the prepared glass slide immediately using a flat curved spreading movement and not a rubbing circular one as this could damage the cells. The slide should then be placed flat and flooded with cytology fixative immediately to prevent air-drying and to preserve the cells on the slide. When dry it is placed into a marked slide holder and sent to the cytology laboratory with the completed cervical smear cytology form.

After the smear has been taken, provided no other GUM tests are required, the speculum is removed. The patient is returned to an upright position and asked to dress. The patient may have a small blood-stained discharge for a few days after the smear and it should be explained that this is normal. It happens because the cervix has been scraped by the spatula or cytobrush (Chomet & Chomet, 1991) and is very common when ectopy is present, as the exposed columnar cells are fragile and bleed easily when scraped. The whole procedure of taking a smear including counselling the patient normally takes about 15 minutes.

Interpretation of smear results

Peel (1995) notes that occasionally cells which suggest that invasive cancer is present may be seen on cervical smear, and this will be reported as such. However, cytology is only 80% accurate in diagnosing early invasive cancer (Husain, 1990). Equivocal smears, which often result from the cytologist being unable to differentiate between inflammatory changes and mild dyskaryosis, are now reported as borderline rather than using the term atypia that was used before (Peel, 1995). Koilocytosis as a result of HPV infection may be reported. Dyskaryosis is the term used to refer to abnormalities in the nucleus and is graded mild, moderate or severe. Dysplasia is the term that relates to abnormalities of position of cells and is only really used now in relation to a biopsy specimen that shows the position of various types of cells, although in the past dysplasia has been used rather interchangeably with dyskaryosis.

The classification of results is only a guide to the likely pathology and must not be taken as a definite diagnosis (Peel, 1995). False negative results may occur for various reasons:

* if a lesion is small, too few cells to give an adequate sample may have been exfoliated;
* if the smear is too thick or thin or contaminated by too many red blood cells, possibly due to being taken wrongly;
* if the smear is incorrectly stained;
* if the smear was badly taken due to inexperience on the part of the person taking the smear, or if the laboratory personnel who read smears are tired or not properly trained.

Some researchers suggest that women should have a second smear a year after the first to try and reduce the false negative rate. However, Husain (1990) suggests this is unnecessary and wasteful and should only be done if the first smear is taken in a woman over 30 years old. Sometimes false positive smear results can be due to errors in interpreting the result when acute inflammation is present, whether it is caused by bacterial, viral, fungal or protozoal infection. Problems of interpretation may also occur when the epithelium is atrophic due to lack of oestrogen (Peel, 1995).

Experienced GUM nurses can play an important role in providing back-up explanation to patients who may not always understand the doctor's account. Consequently a nurse can refer to the smear report and provide understanding of the following points suggested by Austoker (1994):

1.   A smear showing borderline nuclear or mildly dyskaryotic change is normally repeated 6 months later, as requested by

the cytology service and a colposcopy should be considered only if it is still abnormal.

2.   At least two consecutive negative smears 6 months or more apart are usually required following a borderline or mild dyskaryotic smear before recall can be reduced, ideally to 3-yearly.

3.   Women with moderate or severe dyskaryosis should have a colposcopy straight away on the cytologist's recommendation.

4.   Women with HPV are followed up according to the CIN grade that is found and not just because they have HPV. This is particularly important in GUM where so many patients have HPV.

Austoker (1994) notes that although the consensus of opinion is that a patient with a single mildly dyskaryotic smear should have a repeat smear 6 months later and be referred for colposcopy only if there is persistent dyskaryosis, some clinicians believe that women with such smears should be colposcoped immediately. This recommendation is made because a small proportion of smears showing mild dyskaryosis will progress to severe dyskaryosis, although most will revert to normal or persist as mild dyskaryosis. Colposcopy is recommended when moderate or severe dyskaryosis is found on a smear.

Chomet and Chomet (1991) note various other reports and recommendations that may be made on cytology results. Actinomycetes are fungi that are often found when a woman has an IUD in place. They do not cause cervical cancer and normal recall is advised. If a smear has been air dried, the cells are inadequately fixed and a repeat smear is needed. An atrophic smear normally reflects the low oestrogen levels found in post-menopausal women and normal recall is advised. Atypia or atypical cells show very mild cellular changes and a repeat smear is advised within 6 months. Colposcopy is normally recommended if cellular changes continue. HPV results in koilocytic cells being present and is often accompanied by mild, moderate or severe dyskaryosis. *Trichomonas vaginalis* (TV) may cause inflammatory cells on cervical cytology and should be treated. A repeat smear may be taken 3–6 months later.

If inflammatory changes are reported on cytology it is important to take a repeat smear after 3–6 months, and if the inflammation persists colposcopy is usually advised to exclude underlying CIN. When a smear is reported as inflammatory, McGarry (1991) suggests that a repeat smear is taken 2 months after appropriate treatment has been given.

Taking a good smear

Chomet and Chomet (1991) suggest that sometimes it may be difficult to take a good smear from women who have had procedures
carried out on their cervix, for example removal of CIN by
diathermy, cryotherapy or cone biopsy. This is because such procedures occasionally lead to stenosis of the endocervical canal and the
SCJ and transformation zone being moved up into the cervical
canal, which make it difficult to obtain a good sample. However, Peel
(1995) believes that such problems are greatly reduced by the use of
local methods such as cryotherapy and diathermy rather than cone
biopsy. If a woman has had an episiotomy or been stitched following
childbirth, the cervix may be distorted making it difficult to take a
smear (Chomet & Chomet, 1991).

During pregnancy the cervix undergoes certain changes that can
last up to 3 months after delivery. It is safe to take smears during
pregnancy, though smears taken at this time may not have endocervical cells in them or they may show only postnatal changes. Peel
(1995) notes that cancer of the cervix is found in one in 2 000–5 000
pregnancies and as cytology is routinely done at the first antenatal
visit, up to 80% of cervical cancer in pregnancy is diagnosed during
the first 6 months of the pregnancy.

It has been noted that the presence of endocervical cells may be
used as a criteria for good smears. Macgregor (1991) notes that the
presence of endocervical cells shows that the cervix has been visualised, but if a smear is taken from high in the cervical canal it may
only show endocervical cells and it will not be able to detect cancer
in the transformation zone. Where ectopy is present, it is fairly easy
to get endocervical cells on a smear (Macgregor, 1991). Husain
(1990) notes that it is important to get a representative sample and
Austoker (1994) says that it is the responsibility of the person taking
the smear to make sure the cervix has been adequately sampled.
Austoker (1994) also believes that smears should ideally contain
endocervical cells, metaplastic cells, squamous cells and endocervical mucus and that adequate smears should contain squamous cells
and two out of three of the other cells or mucus. In Avon, the cervical
cytology course requires nurses to have the presence of endocervical
cells reported on at least 50% of the smears they have taken to obtain
a pass for the course (Robbins, 1994).

Various different types of spatulas have been used to take smears
over the years. Bauman (1993) notes that the wooden spatula
designed by Ayre in the 1940s has been modified a number of times

and that plastic spatulas have also been made. Wolfendale et al. (1987) tested the Aylesbury spatula against the Ayre spatula in a study of 17 000 smears. They reported a better cell content in smears in all age groups and 22% more smears diagnosing dyskaryosis when the Aylesbury spatula was used. Work done by Woodman et al. (1991) found that using a Rocket spatula rather than an Ayre spatula was more likely to produce a smear containing endocervical cells and less likely to show immature metaplastic cells, but that the proportion of dyskaryosis found was about equal with both spatulas.

A newer development is that of the cervical brush. Husain (1990) suggests that it is useful to take an additional sample with an endocervical brush, particularly if the woman has a narrow cervical os. He also explains that a brush is rolled onto the slide, rather than rubbed, to get the specimen. An analysis of various trials of spatulas and brushes was carried out by Bauman (1993) and she concluded that using a cervical brush for cervical smears has a significant impact on the sampling of endocervical cells, though whether this improved the diagnosis of dyskaryosis was not clear. She also suggested that although brushes are more expensive, they may be more cost effective in the long term, but that no instrument will always give perfect smears.

Conclusion

Although using different types of spatulas may have an impact on smear taking, the person taking the smear is more important than the spatula type (Macgregor, 1991). It is crucial that nurses in GUM give patients good explanations and information about smear results particularly about abnormal results. Austoker (1994) states that women given results of abnormal smears are often very anxious, that written information is often very useful for women and that information should be easy to read.

McKie (1993) notes that women who have a smear are looking for reassurance and insurance, while health professionals see screening as a control and surveillance measure for cervical cancer.

Overall, training for taking smears is one of the most important issues for nurses. Robbins (1994) notes that there are many advantages to having more reliable, competent smear takers who are not GPs and that many women would prefer another woman to take their smears.

GUM nurses should be able to offer patients the choice of having a smear taken by a woman if no female doctor is available and ensure that good samples are taken with a full explanation, encouraging the patient to return for repeat smears if necessary.

Colposcopy

Introduction

Colposcopy was first described by Hans Hinselmann, who invented the colposcope in 1925. He devised an instrument that incorporated an ordinary microscope, modified to provide binocular vision and illumination, and which was mounted on a movable arm to facilitate easy, sensitive control. To achieve a clear view of the cervix he used a speculum inserted into the vagina and opened to show the cervix. He thought that cervical cancer might start as small ulcers or tumours that could be detected if the area was magnified (Chomet & Chomet, 1991). Evans (1990) notes that magnification of 5–15 diameters (times) is all that is needed for colposcopy. Hinselmann spent a lot of time examining the cervices of women using the colposcope. Evans (1990) notes that Hinselmann discovered the effect of various solutions, such as acetic acid, which brings out abnormal areas on the cervix as white patches. He also found that Lugol's iodine stains normal cervical and vaginal epithelium brown when applied to the cervix; this is known as the Schiller's test (Chomet & Chomet, 1991).

For many years, colposcopy was used mainly in German-speaking countries; it was only after the Second World War that Hinselmann travelled to South America and the technique of colposcopy became more widespread (Chomet & Chomet, 1991).

Cytology and colposcopy are complementary methods of diagnosing cervical abnormalities, the former laboratory and the latter clinical (Kolstad & Stafl, 1982). Colposcopy is a relatively new diagnostic procedure in Britain, but with the detection of cervical abnormalities by cytology and then colposcopic detection, accurate diagnosing and early treatment is much easier. Evans (1990) suggests that there should be a colposcope in every GUM clinic, as colposcopy is essential when examining patients in GUM. British gynaecologists became interested in colposcopy in the 1960s and set up the British Colposcopy Group (now the British Society for Colposcopy and Cervical Pathology, BSCCP) in 1971 (Chomet & Chomet, 1991).

There is no doubt that colposcopy is of great value, not only in the diagnosis, management and follow-up of early cancerous lesions of the cervix but also in the evaluation and treatment of benign conditions.

Colposcopy has become much more popular as pre-cancers are occurring in younger women in whom the early diagnosis of abnormality is essential to allow the use of local treatment which reduces the need for surgery, such as hysterectomy, and so maintains the patient's chance of pregnancy and childbirth (Chomet & Chomet, 1991).

Indications for colposcopy

CIN may be suspected in patients with abnormal cervical cytology but the diagnosis and treatment will depend on referral of such women for colposcopic assessment. Evans (1990) suggests that women with dyskaryosis on cervical smear provide the majority of patients for colposcopy. He notes that because of the connection between HPV and cervical abnormalities, all patients with present or previous warts or whose partners have or have had warts should have a colposcopy. Evans (1990) also suggests that women with persistent inflammatory smears following treatment should also be colposcoped.

However, the recommendation in relation to HPV infection is summed up by Anderson (1993) who states that in the UK, a woman who has HPV but has not had dyskaryosis on a smear result should not be routinely colposcoped. Treatment of women with HPV should be managed according to the grade of CIN found on smear, not just because HPV is present (Duncan, 1993).

Patients who are referred for colposcopy are those who have an abnormal cytology result: persistent borderline nuclear changes or mild dyskaryosis; moderate or severe dyskaryosis when it is first reported on a smear; glandular abnormalities; or if invasive cancer is suggested by the smear report (Anderson, 1993). In addition Soutter (1993) states that if there is any suspicion of cancer on clinical examination the woman should have a colposcopy regardless of what is reported on the smear.

Preparing the patient

Preparation of a woman for colposcopy should have been started when the cervical smear was taken. Roberts and Blunt (1994) note that giving full and accurate information about abnormal cytology results at the time a smear is taken can reduce anxiety levels should such results occur. Nugent and Tamlyn-Leaman (1992) found in their study of what women knew about colposcopy, that 32% did not know why colposcopy was done. They found that women wanted information before their colposcopy appointment and they suggest that nurses in colposcopy clinics should develop information packs. Soutter (1993) emphasises how important it is to explain that it is not cancer that is being looked for but changes that might perhaps turn into cancer in 10–20 years' time. This explanation can reduce worry caused by an abnormal smear result.

McGarry (1991) states that a woman should be told that colposcopy normally takes 10–15 minutes, that there may be some bleeding afterwards, that colposcopy without treatment being carried out is painless and that colposcopy can, if necessary, be undertaken when a woman is menstruating. Chomet and Chomet (1991) feel that a woman is more sensitive vaginally during her period and so this time should be avoided if possible. Cartier (1993) advises that colposcopy is best carried out between days 8 and 12 of a woman's normal cycle when there is the most mucus and the cervical os is most widely dilated. However, women on the contraceptive pill have thick mucus throughout the cycle.

Colposcopy can be carried out during pregnancy (Chomet & Chomet, 1991), though Cartier (1993) notes that it is always a long procedure and can be difficult at this time. Rickert et al. (1994) looked at ways of reducing anxiety and related body movement during colposcopy in younger women and found that watching a music video, rather than watching the procedure on the monitor or not watching anything, helped reduce body movement.

The colposcopy procedure and findings

The patient is examined in a similar position to that used for a smear, though most GUM clinics use a gynae couch that allows the patient to be in the lithotomy position during the examination. It can be helpful to have nurses available, not only to assist the colposcopist but to reassure and care for the patient (Chomet & Chomet, 1991). Table 2.2 lists the equipment needed for colposcopy. It is important to examine the whole genital area. Soutter (1993) suggests that a careful bi-manual examination is done at this point, touching the end of the cervix as little as possible. Chomet and Chomet (1991) note that the vulva and vagina should be checked first, particularly to see if any warts are present.

A bi-valve speculum is then inserted into the vagina. Evans (1990) notes that the use of a broad-bladed speculum is important to allow good visualisation of the vaginal fornices as well as the cervix.

Table 2.2: Equipment for colposcopy

- gloves
- speculae of various sizes, warmed if metal
- sponge forceps
- cotton wool/cotton bud/colpettes
- colposcope
- histology pots containing formalin and histology forms
- endocervical speculum
- biopsy forceps
- needle (to remove tissue from the jaws of the biopsy forceps)
- acetic acid 3 or 5%
- Lugol's solution or similar iodine preparation
- caustic applicator such as 75% silver nitrate or 25% potassium nitrate
- sanitary pad

A cervical smear may be taken at this stage (Soutter, 1993), though Cartier (1993) feels it is better not to do a smear at colposcopy, as bleeding may obscure the area and make examination difficult. Evans (1990) suggests that other GUM tests for TV, candida or herpes may be taken if indicated clinically.

Saline is then used to clean the cervix and vagina. At this point it is possible to see leukoplakia, surface and vascular changes and condylomata acuminata, if they are present (Soutter, 1993).

Leukoplakia

Leukoplakia or 'white patch' was of great interest to Hinselmann when he first started to undertake colposcopy (Kolstad & Stafl, 1982). It is thick, white epithelium which is visible if there is a thick keratin layer (Cartier, 1993). True leukoplakia is visible before acetic acid is applied to the cervix and should be identified at this stage. It is important to biopsy the area of leukoplakia as it can obscure under-lying disease of the cervix (Soutter, 1993).

Surface and vascular changes

Invasive cancer may be recognised by the distortion of the surface of the cervix and may be diagnosed after saline has cleared away any overlying mucus (Soutter, 1993). Chomet and Chomet (1991) note that the application of saline makes the vascular pattern easier to see and the appearance of blood vessels should be noted. Invasive lesions have irregular blood vessels on them, often looking like corkscrews or commas and instead of branches getting smaller, vessels which are tributaries are often the same size as the main vessels (Soutter, 1993). Kolstad and Stafl (1982) note that this is referred to as punctation and that it is normally only found in an area that is clearly demarcated. They also describe a vascular pattern called mosaic and again this is found in well defined areas. Sometimes the pattern is so irregular that it is referred to just as atypical vessels.

Condylomata acuminatum

Condylomas are papillomatous tumours or warts, either flat or more distinctly condylomatus or fleshy. They are normally recognised by their surface, which is frond-like and regular, and Soutter (1993) suggests a biopsy should be taken, particularly if they are seen on the transformation zone, as they are not always benign.

The next stage in colposcopy is the application of 3–5% acetic acid to the cervix. Chomet and Chomet (1991) suggest that this may cause a short stinging sensation to the woman and that abnormalities that were previously unseen appear as areas of different degrees of whiteness, pattern and texture. There are many normal changes that can be identified after the application of acetic acid. Evans (1990) notes that the whitening effect develops quicker and fades quicker in thin epithelium such as columnar epithelium and is slower to develop but lasts longer in thicker epithelium such as squamous epithelium. Normal squamous epithelium is a regular pink colour on a smooth surface, though Nabothian follicles may be present, while normal columnar epithelium has villi or folds and will go white very quickly for a short time only before returning to its red colour (Soutter, 1993). Cartier (1993) notes that the SCJ appears very quickly with acetic acid and it has a clear edge of squamous epithelium (Soutter, 1993). Endocervical polyps may also be seen and atrophic epithelium may appear slightly acetowhite (Soutter, 1993).

Acetowhite epithelium

Acetowhite epithelium may occur in normal epithelium as well as abnormal and the density of the nuclei in the epithelium determines the colour formed by acetic acid (Soutter, 1993). Evans (1990) states that acetowhite epithelium occurs where there is squamous metaplasia with immature squamous epithelium and in non-condylomatus wart virus infection, and both metaplastic and viral lesions normally have irregular edges, with viral lesions sometimes having satellite lesions away from the main area (Soutter, 1993). Metaplastic epithelium tends to have a faint white colour. Evans (1990) goes on to state that acetowhite is found in dysplastic epithelium in the transformation zone, in adenocarcinoma and where inflammation is present. Soutter (1993) explains that CIN usually appears as a thick white colour because there are a lot of closely packed, well nucleated cells, though a thin area of CIN III may be as faint a colour as metaplasia. Also CIN normally has clear, well marked edges. It is important that the edge of an acetowhite lesion is seen at the SCJ. Cartier (1993) notes that if the SCJ is in the endocervical canal, endocervical forceps such as Kogans or des Jardins may be needed to open up the canal, or a cotton swab may be used instead. If the whole lesion cannot be seen, then the colposcopy must be reported as unsatisfactory or incomplete (Soutter, 1993) and a cone biopsy should be carried out to determine the extent of the lesion (Chomet & Chomet, 1991). Soutter (1993) notes that vascular patterns such as mosaic and punctation may be seen at this stage as well as before the application of acetic acid.

The next stage in the colposcopy may be the use of iodine to perform the Schiller's test.

The Schiller's test

Iodine, normally in the form of Lugol's solution, is painted on the cervix and vagina (Cartier, 1993). Chomet and Chomet (1991) explain that cells containing glycogen stain brown when iodine is applied and as normal squamous epithelium contains glycogen, it stains brown. Immature metaplasia, normal endocervical epithelium, sometimes atrophic epithelium and abnormal areas such as CIN do not stain brown with the Schiller's test. The SCJ must also be painted with iodine. Iodine and acetic acid are both used to diagnose CIN and other abnormalities (Chomet & Chomet, 1991).

Colposcopy may be used to help diagnose CIN. An expert colposcopist can then decide where to take a biopsy from and what type of biopsy to take or what procedure to undertake. Soutter (1993) notes that the cytology report, findings at colposcopy and the histological result of a punch biopsy are used in combination to make a diagnosis.

Biopsy findings

CIN is used to describe pre-cancerous change that has not developed further than the cervical epithelium and it covers the range of abnormality from mild dyskaryosis to carcinoma in situ.

Although Husain (1990) suggests that up to 70% of CIN I cases will revert to normal, which is why a first smear showing mild dyskaryosis should be repeated 3–6 months later before colposcopy is undertaken, Soutter (1993) believes that about 20% of CIN I–II lesions will progress to CIN III within 2 years.

Table 2.3 shows the various ways of classifying dyskaryosis and CIN. Ulmer (1994) and Evans (1990) relate CIN to dysplasia or dyskaryosis, whereas Chomet and Chomet (1991) note that some centres refer to smears by class numbered from 1–5.

Table 2.3: Classification of CIN

Class	Negative smears	Dyskaryosis	CIN/dysplasia
Class I	Normal		
Class II	Inflammatory changes Squamous metaplasia		
Class III		Mild	Mild dysplasia CIN I
Class IV		Moderate	Moderate dysplasia CIN II
Class V		Severe	Severe dysplasia eg. carcinoma in situ CIN III

Procedures and treatments at colposcopy

Various treatments and procedures may be carried out at colposcopy depending on the equipment available, the policy of the clinic and colposcopist, and the degree of abnormality seen during colposcopy. Some clinics routinely undertake punch biopsy and then bring the woman back for further treatment or refer them to a gynaecologist for outpatient or inpatient treatment. Other clinics use loop diathermy to obtain a biopsy specimen and undertake treatment at the same procedure. Treatments work either by destroying or ablating cells or by excising or removing abnormal tissue (Soutter, 1993). Such treatments are normally very successful in getting rid of disease while maintaining the structure and function of the cervix. Some of the procedures and treatments that may be carried out in the GUM setting are described below. It is important to remember that whatever method is used to remove CIN, the skill and knowledge of the operator is paramount.

Cervical punch biopsy

A punch biopsy involves a small piece of tissue being taken from an abnormal area and sent to histology for examination (Chomet & Chomet, 1991). As a punch biopsy samples the layers of epithelium it will show whether a pre-cancer has invaded through the layers (Soutter, 1993). Chomet and Chomet (1991) suggest that a punch biopsy does not hurt a woman as such a small sample is taken and the cervix does not have much sensation of pain. However Soutter (1993) stresses the need for sharp instruments otherwise pain may be caused. Some problems of punch biopsy are that the severity of the lesion may not be recognised or the biopsy may not sample the abnormal area properly (Soutter, 1993; Chomet & Chomet, 1991). Silver nitrate sticks may be used to stop any bleeding after the biopsy has been taken.

Loop diathermy

This procedure is known as large loop excision of the transformation zone (LLETZ) and some clinics use it to obtain a biopsy rather than taking a punch biopsy. Prendiville (1993) explains that LLETZ was developed to provide an alternative to cone biopsy and destructive methods of treating the cervix and the aim was to completely remove the transformation zone. Soutter (1993) states that if there is any suggestion of invasive disease, then only a loop biopsy should be done and not excision of the full transformation zone.

The LLETZ technique uses a thin wire loop, which has an electric current passed through it from a monopolar electrosurgical unit, to excise a sample of tissue while a smoke evacuator unit is used (Soutter, 1993; Chomet & Chomet, 1991). Prendiville (1993) points out that taking a small loop biopsy produces a much better quality biopsy than the use of punch biopsy forceps. Unlike a cone biopsy, LLETZ is an outpatient procedure carried out under local anaesthetic. Although lignocaine, either with or without adrenaline, is often used for local anaesthesia, Prendiville (1993) advises the use of citanest with octapressin through a dental needle and syringe.

The electrosurgical unit gives a blend of cutting and coagulating diathermy, which cuts out the specimen and stops bleeding at the same time (Ulmer, 1994), therefore there is not much bleeding. The ideal in this technique is for the operator to have a steady hand so the wire is passed slowly and smoothly through the tissue of the cervix allowing the wire to form a steam envelope around itself, producing a good specimen with no drying heat damage to it (Prendiville, 1993). Ulmer (1994) states that LLETZ is a quick procedure, as effective as laser treatment and less expensive. As LLETZ is often performed as a treatment at the first colposcopy as well as for obtaining a biopsy, the patient avoids an anxious wait for a biopsy result and later treatment (Roberts & Blunt, 1994).

After the specimen has been taken, the cervix is checked and light coagulation diathermy using a ball electrode is applied to any bleeding points (Prendiville, 1993). Soutter (1993) notes only a small percentage of post-procedure problems apart from vaginal discharge, which normally lasts no more than 2 weeks.

Cold coagulation

Evans (1990) notes that cold coagulation as an ablative treatment of CIN has produced some good results and Chomet and Chomet (1991) suggest a 95% cure rate for CIN III with this treatment. The probe used is heated to 100°C or just above the boiling point of water and this is termed cold coagulation in comparison to diathermy, which may produce temperatures of up to 1500°C (Evans, 1990; Soutter, 1993). The probe is applied for 20 seconds at a time in overlapping applications to the transformation zone (Soutter, 1993), and McGarry (1991) suggests four applications are normally needed. Soutter (1993) notes that it is important not to touch the vagina with the probe and where there are large areas on the vagina this procedure is difficult. Patients may get a heavy discharge, which leads some operators to prescribe sultrin cream for use post-procedure, and some women may have some crampy pain but this treatment can be done without a general anaesthetic (Chomet & Chomet, 1991; Soutter, 1993).

Cryotherapy

Cryotherapy is a popular form of ablative treatment for CIN. However, many commentators suggest that it should only be used for small areas of CIN I or II, as tissue is generally destroyed to a depth of only 5 mm and rarely to 8 mm which may not be adequate for larger lesions (Chomet & Chomet, 1991; Soutter, 1993). Evans (1990) is a great advocate of cryotherapy and describes how nitrous oxide gas expanding under pressure through a small hole in the probe produces a freezing effect of –30°C. Carbon dioxide may also be used and delivered through a gun pipe unit in the same way

(Chomet & Chomet, 1991) or liquid nitrogen may be used. Evans (1990) suggests a double freeze technique of 2 minutes each freeze with a thaw in between and some operators use lubricating jelly on the area to be treated to improve the contact (Soutter, 1993). There is normally a heavy watery discharge for 2–3 weeks after the procedure and some women may have a foul-smelling discharge, such as that experienced with bacterial vaginosis, from the treated area necrosing; this can be treated with metronidazole (Evans, 1990). This method of treating CIN can be carried out as an outpatient procedure with no anaesthetic and only minor side effects such as cramp-like pain and faintness are noted (Chomet & Chomet, 1991). This treatment is widely available, but care must be taken to select suitable lesions for treatment (Soutter, 1993).

Carbon dioxide laser

Evans (1990) notes that evaporation of tissue by carbon dioxide laser is very effective and can be accurately controlled. Carbon dioxide is turned into energy within the laser and this energy, when beamed at tissues, is absorbed by the intracellular fluid. This causes the fluid to boil and the tissue to be vaporised (Soutter, 1993; Peel, 1995). The smoke produced must be extracted by suction applied directly to a special tube on the speculum. Laser evaporation is done under colposcopic control and care must be taken to avoid thermal damage to healthy tissue because although the thermal effect does stop bleeding at the site, if a laser is used to excise CIN and so obtain a specimen for histology, the thermal effect can also distort the tissue (Soutter, 1993; Ulmer, 1994).

The destruction caused by laser must reach a depth of 5–7mm to ensure that all the cells involved, particularly glands, are destroyed (Peel, 1995). Most operators use a local anaesthetic to ensure patients do not feel any discomfort and there appear to be very few post-operative complications and good healing occurs with this method (Chomet & Chomet, 1991; Peel, 1995). Soutter (1993) notes that many patients will have a small amount of discharge for up to 10 days and suggests using sultrin cream for a week. It has been shown that treatment by laser is very effective with 95% of patients treated found to be free of further disease after one year (Chomet & Chomet, 1991).

Peel (1995) notes that a laser can be used to take a cone biopsy, instead of a routine knife cone biopsy, and that this can be done as an outpatient procedure. However, this is not routinely done in GUM clinics. The main disadvantages of laser treatment are that it is very expensive to buy the equipment and running costs are high. Soutter (1993) notes along with many others, that when comparing laser with LLETZ as an excisional treatment, LLETZ is both quicker and much less expensive.

Further inpatient treatments and procedures

There are other treatments for CIN and invasive cancer of the cervix that are done as inpatient procedures with a general anaesthetic.

Electrodiathermy or cautery

Although Soutter (1993) suggests that diathermy to ablate CIN can be carried out as an outpatient with very good local anaesthesia, many people believe this procedure is too painful without general anaesthesia (Evans, 1990).

Cone biopsy

As has been noted previously, cone biopsy should be performed if the CIN lesion has not been completely seen at colposcopy. Peel (1995) also states that if invasive cancer is suspected or if positive smears have been reported following a normal colposcopy, then a cone biopsy should be carried out. Soutter (1993) reports that cone biopsy should not replace colposcopy and that a woman should be colposcoped in the operating theatre before the cone biopsy is performed. As with all treatments for CIN, the amount of tissue removed by cone biopsy will depend on the extent of the lesion and ideally there will be a margin of normal tissue in the cone, showing that the abnormality has been fully excised (Chomet & Chomet, 1991). There can be complications to cone biopsy, such as haemorrhage and later cervical stenosis, especially as nowadays cone biopsy is usually only performed on women with more difficult problems (Soutter, 1993). Laser cone biopsy may be an alternative, as previously discussed.

Hysterectomy

A radical Wertheim's hysterectomy including removal of the uterus, cervix, tubes, ovaries, lymph nodes and surrounding tissue may be advised where there is deep invasive cancer or involvement of the lymph system (McGarry, 1991).

Information and follow-up for patients following colposcopy and procedures

Most patients worry about intercourse, future contraception, pregnancy and the use of tampons. It is important that the nurse gives the patient good information to allay any uncertainties and worries. Advice given differs from clinic to clinic, but a guide is that if a biopsy or treatment has been performed, then intercourse should be avoided for 4–6 weeks, tampons should not be used for a similar period and the patient should take it easy for the rest of the day. It is important to stress that, depending on the treatment given, some discharge is normal for up to 2 weeks, but if heavy bleeding, irritation or pain occurs the patient should return to the clinic urgently or go to her GP or casualty department if the GUM clinic is closed. Haemorrhage or infection following colposcopic procedures are not common but can be serious if left untreated. Chomet and Chomet (1991) advise that swimming and hot baths are best avoided for a week after a biopsy has been taken.

If no treatment has been carried out but a biopsy has been taken then the patient should be seen 1–2 weeks later to discuss the results of the biopsy and arrange further treatment. If ablative treatment has been performed many doctors arrange for the patient to return 6 months later for repeat cytology and/or colposcopy.

It is not possible to overemphasise the importance of regular follow-up after colposcopy, abnormal cytology or treatment. Soutter (1993) notes that many recurrences occur more than one year after treatment for CIN, particularly where there is invasive recurrence. Most operators advise that a smear should be taken 4–6 months after treatment and if that is normal then it should be repeated at 12 months and then annually for up to 5–10 years before returning to 3-yearly screening or continuing on annual screening regardless of whether the woman has sex or not (Chomet & Chomet, 1991; Soutter, 1993; Duncan, 1993). The nurse should explain the need for follow-up to the woman following colposcopy and treatment in the GUM clinic and should allow the patient the choice of continuing to have smears taken in the clinic or returning to her GP for them.

Conclusion

Chomet and Chomet (1991) point out that out of every 1 000 women who have a smear done only 1–2 will have invasive cancer and only 1 in 300 women who have a positive smear result will have invasive cancer.

GUM nurses can provide better care for patients by ensuring they have the information they need about their smear or colposcopy. This means giving basic information about female anatomy as well as about smear results and what a colposcopy is (Nugent & Tamlyn-Leamen, 1992). Duncan (1993) advises that verbal and written information given before and after cervical screening and before, during and after colposcopy and treatment reduces anxiety in women.

Trained, knowledgeable GUM nurses are in a key position to answer patients' questions, to provide information and to give reassurance and advice.

References

Anderson M (1993) Selection of patients for treatment – the British view. In Prendiville W (Ed), Large Loop Excision of the Transformation Zone – A Practical Guide to LLETZ. London: Chapman & Hall.

Austoker J (1994) Screening for cervical cancer. British Medical Journal 309: 241–8.

Barton SE, Maddox PH, Jenkins D, Edwards R, Cuzick J, Singer A (1988) Effect of cigarette smoking on cervical epithelial immunity: a mechanism for neoplastic change? Lancet September 17: 652–4.

Bauman BJ (1993) Use of a cervical brush for Papanicolaou smear collection – a meta-analysis. Journal of Nurse-Midwifery 38(5): 267–75.

Cartier R (1993) Principles of competent colposcopic examination. In Prendiville W (Ed), Large Loop Excision of the Transformation Zone – A Practical Guide to LLETZ. London: Chapman & Hall.

Chomet J, Chomet J (1991) Smear Tests. London: Thorsons.

DOH (1993) The Health of the Nation: Key Area Handbook Cancers. London: HMSO.

DOH (1995) Sexually transmitted diseases, England 1994. Department of Health Statistical Bulletin. London: HMSO.

Duncan I (1993) NHS cervical screening programme; guidelines for clinical practice and programme management. In Prendiville W (Ed), Large Loop Excision of the Transformation Zone – A Practical Guide to LLETZ. London: Chapman & Hall.

Evans BA (1990) Colposcopy. In Csonka GW, Oates JK (Eds), Sexually Transmitted Diseases – A Textbook of Genitourinary Medicine. London: Baillière Tindall.

Farlow E (1993) The cervical smear a simple test can save a woman's life. The British Journal of Theatre Nursing 2(11): 4–7.

Hare J (1990) Contraception and sexually transmitted disease. In Csonka GW, Oates JK (Eds), Sexually Transmitted Diseases – A Textbook of Genitourinary Medicine. London: Baillière Tindall.

Held JL (1995) Preventing cervical cancer. Nursing95 25(2): 24.

Hope-Stone HF (1990) Genital malignancies. In Csonka GW, Oates JK (Eds), Sexually Transmitted Diseases – A Textbook of Genitourinary Medicine. London: Baillière Tindall.

Husain OAN (1990) Cervical cytology. In Csonka GW, Oates JK (Eds), Sexually Transmitted Diseases – A Textbook of Genitourinary Medicine. London: Baillière Tindall.

IARC Working Group on Evaluation of Cervical Cancer Screening Programmes (1986) Screening for squamous cervical cancer: duration of low risk after negative results of cervical cytology and its implication for screening policies. British Medical Journal 293: 659–64.

Kolstad P, Stafl A (1982) Atlas of Colposcopy, 3rd edn. Oslo: Universitetsforlaget.

Macgregor JE (1991) What constitutes an adequate cervical smear? British Journal of Obstetrics and Gynaecology 98(1): 6–7.

McGarry J (1991) The cervical smear: 4. Practice Nurse 4(5): 301–4.

McKie L (1993) Women's views of the cervical smear test; implications for nursing practice – women who have had a smear test. Journal of Advanced Nursing 18(8): 1228–34.

Mela H (1993) Prevention of carcinoma of the cervix. Update August 15: 199–200.

Milburn K, MacAskill S (1994) Cervical screening: continuing concerns in the 1990s. Health Education Journal 53(2): 201–13.

Nugent LS, Tamlyn-Leaman K (1992) The colposcopy experience: what do women know? Journal of Advanced Nursing 17(4): 514–20.

Papanicolaou GN, Traut HF (1941) The diagnostic value of vaginal smears in carcinoma of the uterus. American Journal of Obstetrics and Gynecology 42(2): 193–205.

Peel KR (1995) Premalignant and malignant disease of the cervix. In Whitfield CR (Ed), Dewhurst's Textbook of Obstetrics and Gynaecology for Postgraduates, 5th edn. Oxford: Blackwell Science.

Prendiville W (1993) Large loop excision of the transformation zone. In Prendiville W (Ed), Large Loop Excision of the Transformation Zone – A Practical Guide to LLETZ. London: Chapman & Hall.

Rickert VI, Kozlowski KJ, Warren AM, Hendon A, Davis P (1994) Adolescents and colposcopy: the use of different procedures to reduce anxiety. American Journal of Obstetrics and Gynecology February: 504–8.

Robbins S (1994) Taking a better smear. Practice Nurse June 15–30: 18–23.

Roberts RA, Blunt SM (1994) The psychological reaction of women to a colposcopy clinic. British Journal of Obstetrics and Gynaecology 101 September: 751–2.

Soutter P (1993) A Practical Guide to Colposcopy. Oxford: Oxford University Press.

Ulmer BC (1994) Cervical intraepithelial neoplasia. AORN Journal 59(4): 851–60.

Wolfendale MR, Howe-Guest R, Usherwood MMcD, Draper GJ (1987) Controlled trial of a new cervical spatula. British Medical Journal 294: 33–5.

Woodman CJB, Yates M, Williams DR, Ward K, Jordan J, Luesley D (1991) A randomized control trial of two cervical spatulas. British Journal of Obstetrics and Gynaecology 98: 21–4.

Bibliography

Gath DH, Hallam N, Mynors-Wallis L, Day A, Bond SAK (1995) Emotional reactions in women attending a UK colposcopy clinic. The Journal of Epidemiology and Community Health 49: 79–83.

Schnell JD (1975) Cytology and Microbiology of the Vagina. Basel: S Karger.
Skelton S (1991) Cervical smear call and recall. Practice Nurse 3(11): 611–18.

THE LIBRARY
KENT & ... HOSPITAL
TUNBRIDGE WELLS
KENT TN4 8AT

Chapter 3
Contact tracing and patient education

Maureen Baker

Contact tracing

During the First World War, the dramatic increase in the incidence of syphilis and gonorrhoea led to a national network of Special Clinics being set up to deal with the demand for care and to try and arrest the spread of infection by contact tracing and treating sexual partners. Contact tracing may be referred to as partner notification in some clinics. For the purpose of this chapter, the author will use the term contact tracing.

Since the report of the 1916 *Royal Commission on Venereal Disease*, these clinics have undergone various changes of legislation. Until 1948 they were under the control of the local authorities. Since then, they have been taken over by the National Health Service and renamed departments of genito-urinary medicine (GUM). As part of the government's *The Health of the Nation* policy (DOH, 1993) a further change to the name may be introduced to encompass family planning, combining the two specialities under the title of Sexual Health Clinics. A co-ordinated approach such as this would ensure that patients have access to a service in which nursing and medical staff have knowledge of and confidence in both settings (Stedman & Elstein, 1995).

Sexually transmitted diseases (STDs) and their control are a major health problem worldwide today. Contact tracing and public education are two important steps towards their control.

History of contact tracing

GUM has achieved a large measure of success in the control of syphilis and gonorrhoea, aided by both increased ease of treatment with newer drugs and a well organised contact tracing service (Evans, 1990). At the beginning of this century, both mortality and morbidity rates from syphilis were high; actual numbers were difficult to establish as there was thought to be considerable underreporting. One of the first areas of concern was the effect of syphilis on the army, where the number of cases was so large as to prove a threat to efficiency. Tracing of contacts was introduced in the form of *The Contagious Diseases Acts* of 1864, 1866 and 1869, in an attempt to control the spread of infection. The Acts allowed for the examination and detention of prostitutes in hospitals. This caused a considerable outcry because of the double standards of morality which condoned sexual activities of men but persecuted women (Robertson, McMillan & Young, 1989). The Acts were finally repealed in 1886, as there was no evidence that the spread of disease was reduced by these measures.

Various other attempts have been made to introduce legislation, but it is still considered that the most effective control measures are the sensitive handling of the patient interview by the person responsible for advising on health education and contact tracing. Robertson, McMillan and Young (1989) state that 'Compulsory measures are inappropriate and the power to use them inevitably changes attitudes of those working in clinics and discourages attendance in those whose need is greatest.' If treated with respect and reassurance on the confidential nature of the service provided, a greater co-operation with patients can be established. Information about sexual contacts is more likely to be given if patience, kindness and tact are used in the interview process, along with a full explanation of the condition and reasons for the need to ensure that partners are seen and offered appropriate examination, testing and, if necessary, treatment.

In considering who is best suited to carrying out this work, adequate training should be a priority, along with the ability to give clear, easily understood explanations of the various conditions. An open mind, good knowledge of STDs and an awareness of the variations in human sexuality are also essential, if credibility is to be maintained.

Reasons for contact tracing

Contact tracing is generally accepted as an essential element in the epidemiological management of all STDs. It has become standard in all GUM clinics to interview patients and encourage the attendance and treatment of all sexual partners. Whether or not this is an effective measure of control is questionable, but until further research into the various approaches produces new guidelines, it must still be considered an important intervention in the investigation and management of all STDs. The objectives are to identify and treat patients, particularly those who may be asymptomatic, to reduce the incidence of reinfections, to prevent the spread of infection within the population and the serious long-term effects of such conditions. Other factors, for instance better health education and health promotion, more knowledge of STDs, free treatment, changes in contraceptive practices and sexual behaviour, may play a larger part in the rise in numbers of people seeking treatment at GUM clinics.

Those working in GUM who are dealing with the sensitive area of sexual health, must also consider the psychological trauma that could be sustained by the partner or partners notified about their possible exposure to STDs. Counselling skills are essential for those working within this field, from the first possible contact with clients either by drop-in to the clinic or by telephone for advice or information. Approaching clients in a non-judgmental, sympathetic manner can reassure and encourage attendance for full examination and treatment and provide the opportunity for education. A sound knowledge of GUM, the conditions, diagnosis, treatment and complications, including hereditary conditions, is required to obtain the full benefits of contact tracing. The special training needs of those undertaking this role should be identified and met to enable the work of contact tracing and patient education to be carried out satisfactorily. The list below is a guide to the qualities and experience required for this demanding work:

1.   Basic counselling skills with special emphasis on relationship counselling and the ability to undertake open discussion on sexuality and sexual behaviour.
2.   Good knowledge of the history of STDs, including human immunodeficiency virus (HIV) infection.
3.   The epidemiology of STDs, particularly transmission and the implications of failure to treat sexual partners. This is particularly important in those conditions that are asymptomatic.
4.   The psychosocial implications of STDs and HIV.
5.   Good communication skills for interviewing and educational skills for teaching.
6.   Sound knowledge of the methods of contact tracing and notification.

7.   Referral to other agencies available when necessary.
8.   Importance of full and accurate record keeping.
9.   Regulations regarding confidentiality.
10.   Ability to evaluate the effectiveness of interviewing and the ability to adapt the work to the resources available and the specific problems within the area of practice.

Process of contact tracing

The process of contact tracing starts following initial examination and testing of a patient, known as the index patient, who presents at the GUM clinic.

At this first interview, counselling should cover the sexual transmissibility of the infection and the risk to partners, who may be asymptomatic; the possibility of re-infection of the index patient if partners are not seen and treated when required; and the health risks to that patient, their future sexual partners and the future partners of their contacts.

These issues are best raised at the time of diagnosis by the health adviser or health care worker who initiates the process of contact tracing. For the purpose of discussion, the contact tracing process can be divided into 'patient referral' and 'provider referral'.

Patient referral

When considering the methods used within patient referral, the most common will be the issue of a contact slip to the index patient. This requires the willingness and co-operation of the patient to give a slip to each of their sexual contacts.

The contact slip should contain details of the hospital of origin, the reference number of the patient and the diagnostic Department of Health code, with the date of attendance at the clinic entered on both the slip and the counterfoil. This is to allow cross-checking in the event of a contact attending another hospital. When this happens, the slip should be returned to the hospital of origin as soon as possible, with the name and address of the hospital where the contact was seen and information on the treatment given.

The reference numbers used in the diagnostic coding of conditions are listed within the contact slip book and follow the Department of Health codes. New codes are issued as required for additional investigations, infections or treatments carried out within the service. When the contact is abroad, these codes do not apply and World Health Organization codes may have to be used. However, these are not widely recognised and in some cases it would be preferable to name the infection. When diagnosis has been made at other centres such as GP surgeries, family planning clinics, hospital outpatient clinics, or when an infection is identified while a person is an inpatient on a hospital ward, the process of contact tracing may not be considered by staff in these areas and treatment given to only the patient presenting with the problem. If referred to a GUM clinic, the contact tracing process can be started.

However, as more doctors in general practice extend their investigations with more readily available and easy to use diagnostic kits, the way forward may be to improve the knowledge of those health care workers who at present have neither the skills to carry out this work nor the necessary protocols in place for control of sexually transmitted conditions. Consideration could be given to the development of a simpler form of contact slip, using a less extensive range of codes, which could be used in GP surgeries. If the doctor is not comfortable with broaching the subject or discussing sexual matters, but is aware of the need to ensure all sexual partners of the patient are treated, referral to a GUM clinic would still be an option. Many patients have difficulty in persuading their partners to attend a GUM clinic, but feel they would respond to a referral to their own GP, so this could have a beneficial effect on limiting the spread of infection. With closer liaison between GPs and the GUM service and the development of a protocol for contact tracing, other than within a GUM clinic, the more open sexual health label could begin to be applied and help to dispel the stigma that is still felt to apply to the GUM service.

Provider referral

There are three methods of provider referral:

1.   Letter – with this, care should be taken to ensure the correct name and address are supplied by the index patient. The envelope should be marked 'Private and confidential' and should not be identifiable as being sent from a hospital. No reference to the specific infection should be made and a telephone number for easy contact with the health adviser or person with whom the contact can discuss the need for attendance, should also be included.

2.   Telephone – before disclosing the reason for the call, the iden-

tity of the patient contact has to be established. This can be difficult and has to be handled in a sensitive way to avoid distress. An interview should be encouraged as soon as possible to discuss the personal nature of the information given to the health care worker.

3.   Home visit – this has the advantage of being able to reassure and counsel the contact about the possible exposure to infection, encouraging attendance for examination and treatment.

These methods of provider referral should be discussed at the initial interview with the index patient and some of the more important associated issues can be raised at this time.

The contact tracing role

It should be remembered that for any one patient attending a clinic, there are at least two other people involved – the person who infected the index patient and the person who infected him/her (Adler, 1990). This presents a challenging prospect to those responsible for undertaking the task of tracing such contacts and ensuring that treatment is given.

The responsibility for contact tracing falls mainly on the health adviser, but it can be undertaken by any member of the team who has the appropriate skills and knowledge of the process to maintain the same standards as the health adviser. The person responsible will vary from one clinic to another. In certain areas, with busy clinics and large numbers of attenders, the recommendation is for one or more health advisers to be employed for the purpose of tracing contacts and advising on sexual health. In other clinics, the nursing staff may be responsible for this once they have been trained to give specialist advice and have developed the appropriate skills.

The examining doctor may issue the contact slips and initiate the process of contact tracing before referring the patient to the health adviser. Some infections have priority over others, in terms of the urgency for informing contacts of a possible exposure. The conditions will be discussed more fully within the relevant chapters of this book, but an example of how this may be approached is shown in Table 3.1.

It should be remembered that where the presenting condition is, for example, genital warts, there is always the possibility of another STD being present and this should be stressed when interviewing the index patient and contacts. When the patient has been given a

Table 3.1: Priority of infections relating to informing contacts

Very high priority	High priority	Recommended
Syphilis	Urethritis	Trichomonas
Gonorrhoea	Chlamydia infection	Candida if recurrent
Hepatitis B	Genital warts	Scabies
	Lymphogranuloma venereum	Molluscum

contact slip for each contact and feels there may be difficulties in presenting these, a time limit could be agreed after which provider referral is initiated if the contact has not presented at a clinic. Good record keeping is essential to ensure that reliable information is stored. It is also important to have a reliable means of cross-referencing so that the return of the contact slips from other clinics can be recorded, along with information on the outcome of screening and treatment of contacts.

In certain instances, it may be more appropriate for contact tracing not to be carried out. This might be in situations where either the index patient or health adviser could be exposed to threats of physical violence. If the contact lives abroad or if there is insufficient information to enable accurate identification to be made, contact tracing would be difficult and in such cases this should be clearly documented in the patient's notes. Some practical aspects surrounding the interview should also be considered, along with the methods used and the person best suited to undertake this work. The interview is a matter of great delicacy, is very time consuming and it must be carried out in privacy if the necessary information is to be obtained (Robertson, McMillan & Young, 1989).

To meet the requirements for time without interruptions and for privacy, a comfortable, quiet room should be available in every clinic. The patient may be very frightened and will require time to understand the information given and the implications of the diagnosis. In some instances, the initial interview could require an hour or longer. A comfortable setting with facilities to provide a cup of tea or coffee and freedom from telephone calls and interruptions will help in the process of allaying fears and anxieties surrounding the diagnosis and will enable fuller discussion on the need to trace sexual partners. Reassurance on the confidentiality of all information disclosed will be a priority when undertaking the contact tracing process.

'All written records must be kept confidential. Where this cannot be ensured, the written records relating to the index case and providing information for locating partners should be destroyed when the partner has been located or it is clear that location will not be possible' (WHO, 1991).

Fear of possible breakdown of relationships will often make it difficult to get sufficient information on the first interview and an appointment should be made for further discussion. Particularly where provider referral has been agreed, the risk of any compromise to confidentiality should be explored. It may be that family or friends are present when a home visit is undertaken. When contact tracing is carried out by the provider, it may be necessary to seek assistance from colleagues in other clinics. A confidential line should be available to facilitate the exchange of information and enable the process of identifying contacts who have attended elsewhere to be documented, along with confirmation of testing, results and treatment. In those conditions where it is essential to trace and treat possible contacts, it may in exceptional circumstances be necessary to apply for a court order. This would only be granted where the courts consider that a person knowingly put others at risk. This will continue to be a debatable point, particularly in relation to the transmission of HIV.

When a patient attends a clinic in response to a contact slip or provider-linked letter, telephone call or home visit, the course of action taken will depend on the seriousness of the condition. Immediate epidemiological treatment may be given following a routine STD screen, on the presumption that the risks indicate the likelihood of infection being present. However, in some circumstances no treatment is given until the results of tests indicate that it is required. In some rare cases, treatment is given without laboratory tests being carried out.

Where cultural barriers exist and contacts refuse to attend for examination, the index patient or a health care worker may be given the treatment to administer to that contact. In this case there is only limited opportunity to counsel or give any health education or health promotion and it is the least acceptable option. Cultural differences may be difficult for the person conducting the interview to appreciate and the index patient can give guidance on any particular beliefs or practices that would affect the adequate screening and treatment required for any particular contact.

Further difficulties may also be experienced with mobile populations such as students at universities, those of no fixed abode or where a temporary accommodation address is given.

Each clinic should have its own protocol for contact tracing and treatment, preferably written to enable all staff to familiarise themselves with the procedure. This could be extended to GP and family planning clinics, where a more general protocol might be introduced to guide all those involved in counselling and screening for STDs, to include criteria for referral to GUM clinics and to ensure partners receive the necessary treatment.

Confidentiality and the legal position

With the government's recommendations in *The Health of the Nation* (DOH, 1993) that the pregnancy rate in under-16s should be halved by the year 2000, special consideration must be given to the careful handling of young people to encourage attendance for examination, treatment and the opportunity to provide good health education and promotion, including contraceptive advice.

Young people's fears that confidentiality may be broken have to be met and they must be reassured that confidentiality is as important when treating under-16s as with anyone else. The examining doctor has to assess the risks to the young person and their ability to understand and consent to any treatment required. This will be particularly important when considering contraceptive advice and possibly administration of the post-coital contraceptive. Counselling for future sexual behaviour and encouragement to involve their parents is important, but priority should be given to establishing a trusting relationship. *Confidentiality and People under 16* offers guidance on how to deal with this issue (BMA et al., undated). Publication of this joint guidance followed the widely publicised Gillick case and clarified the position of those who were unclear about the legal situation in treating patients under 16. Knowledge of this case and the outcome is important to all those working in the field of sexual health and should be extended to include a knowledge of the legal aspects in dealing with crisis intervention required following, for example, an incident of rape. If prosecution is considered, evidence of vaginal penetration is necessary and where children are concerned, there may be difficulty in distinguishing between non-accidental injury and indecent assault. Following rape or indecent assault, fear of having acquired an STD frequently results in early attendance for examination, though it may not be possible to reassure the victim at this stage. However, it will be useful as a means of establishing a baseline for future testing. 'Rape is not an act of sex but an act of violence with sex as the primary weapon' (Craig, 1990). It is very important that all staff bear this in mind when examining victims of rape. Wherever possible the examination should be carried out after full counselling and the choice of a male or female doctor offered. In the case of women, contraception should be discussed. Follow-up appointments should be made for continued counselling and advice. Further tests at a later stage, for example to test for HIV status and hepatitis B, should be offered.

Counselling

In all the situations discussed in this chapter the importance of good counselling skills is paramount and it is important that all staff have knowledge of and skills in counselling. 'Counselling lends itself to many interpretations and can be seen as either a helping relationship or a set of structured activities' (Miller & Bor, 1989).

Counselling skills can be used for:

1.   exploring and managing specific problems;
2.   support and encouragement;
3.   encouraging patients to take responsibility for their own lives and decisions;
4.   crisis intervention.

A counsellor can be considered as an educator, an equal, an encourager or as a catalyst to change. By encouraging patients to look at themselves and their actions, they can be given the guidance they need to enable them to change their lifestyles. By enabling them to talk through their fears and anxieties they can develop more positive approaches to their problems. Good listening skills enable the counsellor to develop a relationship with a patient. The appropriate use of eye contact, body language and voice will make the patient feel they are being listened to and understood and will therefore encourage them to disclose information. 'Good listening entails not only receiving accurately what the other has to say but creating an emotional climate in which people feel safe, free and rewarded for talking' (Nelson-Jones, 1986).

Feedback is important to check that the counsellor has understood what was said. It encourages further exploration and can clear up any misunderstanding. The success of the counselling process will depend on the counsellor responding with understanding to the patient. 'This requires sensitivity, tact and good timing' (Nelson-Jones, 1986).

Allen and Hogg (1993) found that 'health advisers were more likely than medical and nursing staff to talk about counselling in terms of sympathy or acceptance and being non judgmental. The emotional side of counselling was not something with which doctors and nurses appeared particularly familiar or comfortable.' This statement is being overtaken by the improved training available to any health care worker, particularly nurses in GUM, who have an interest in developing the necessary skills to counsel patients. Many are becoming more confident in raising issues surrounding sexually transmitted infection, exploring some of the physical and emotional consequences of conditions and deciding on how best to handle the process of informing sexual partners.

Counselling is a large part of the health education and health promotion processes, but the remainder of this chapter will look more closely at specific issues in relation to patient education within the GUM clinic. Like contact tracing and counselling, an understanding of how people learn and the meaning of the words frequently used but rarely defined, is important in relation to STDs.

Communication

The words communication and learning are used freely, yet the meaning is not always fully understood. Communication could be described as the sending of a message, with feedback necessary to check that the information passed has been understood. Learning is where the message received results in gradual absorption of knowledge with feedback. Alteration of attitude or behaviour may bring about permanent change.

If learning has failed, it could be that communication was not effective or that it was effective but the message was not understood. Feedback is useful as a tool to enable the health educator to identify problem areas.

When communication is mentioned, it is usually thought of in terms of words, that is, verbal communication. This is important but it should be remembered that non-verbal aspects of communication can have a very marked effect on how messages are received.

Facial movements such as smiling or frowning may be the first impression the patient receives and the way they perceive the health professional's attitude towards them can block or open the remainder of the interview process.

Eye contact allows observation of non-verbal messages, sends information and helps to develop exchange in conversations. It is a means of controlling how close the people involved are prepared to get; too much eye contact can be threatening, making patients feel uncomfortable and unable to talk. Listeners look more than talkers and therefore an essential quality in a person involved in the health education process is to be a good listener.

Body movement and gestures will be interpreted as agreement or understanding of what the patient is saying. Posture and body contact can disclose someone's emotional state, e.g. sitting on the edge of the chair, inability to have eye-to-eye contact, restlessness with hand or leg movement, will all indicate extreme anxiety. When a rapport is established, people tend to mirror each other's posture and this can be used to facilitate a more relaxed atmosphere and confidence in the educator. Cultural differences also have to be considered when interpreting such things as gestures and touch. The uses of communication in GUM are summarised in Table 3.2.

Table 3.2: Uses of communication in GUM

1. To allay fears.
2. To minimise psychological effects of the diagnosis of an STD.
3. To bridge the health professional/client relationship.
4. As a manifestation of empathy in times of stress, death or bereavement.
5. As a means of initiating health education.

To communicate effectively with a patient one needs to listen, ask questions, explore a topic, recognise and respond to cues, encourage further conversation and answer questions. In a GUM clinic, the communication process starts at the first patient contact. This is often by telephone and requires special skills to assess the level of anxiety without the benefit of visual body messages and to be able to convey a non-judgmental attitude, to encourage disclosure for a full assessment and/or counselling. Confidentiality may be an area of concern that inhibits disclosure. The reassurance given by a guarantee of confidentiality being preserved may be sufficient to open the conversation.

Patient information

On attendance at a clinic, it is useful to provide patients with information on the service provided and the process of examination for diagnosis of their condition. This information will help prepare the patient for the intimacy of disclosing details about their sexual history and the testing processes used in full screening for STDs. An example of the type of patient information leaflet used for female patients in the author's clinic is shown in Figure 3.1. Following clinical diagnosis, an opportunity is given to discuss the condition and consider the possibility of other STDs being identified when test results become available. Risk reduction will be an important issue at this stage, whether discussing a curable bacterial infection or the implications of a treatable but not curable viral infection. There will be many questions raised at this time, but it may not be possible for patients to fully understand all the information offered. They may be feeling emotional about the need to attend the clinic and the effects a diagnosis of an STD may have on their relationships.

Confidentiality will again be a principal fear of those attending and constant reassurance may be required to enable the best care and treatment to be offered to both client and partner(s).

The form of treatment and possible side effects should be discussed. For example, the possible need for prolonged treatment in

---

CLIENT/INFORMATION SHEET — FEMALE

INTRODUCTION This letter has been prepared to explain how you can gain most benefit from your attendance at the Department of Genito-Urinary Medicine (GUM). This is an out-patient department which specialises in the diagnosis, treatment and counselling of anyone who is worried about sexually transmitted infections and other allied conditions which may affect the fulfilment of a healthy sex life.

CONFIDENTIALITY We would like to reassure you that any personal information given to us will be kept completely confidential and no information will be released to anyone without your consent.

YOUR FIRST VISIT On reporting to the GUM Reception Office you will be asked to wait in the waiting area until the receptionist is available to take you into the office, where she will prepare a numbered file with your personal details such as name and date of birth. You will be asked if we can contact you or your doctor, should this be necessary in the future, and your wishes will be respected as to any contact sources. You will be informed of your personal file number which will be used on tests and for further appointments. You will then be given a number which will identify your file when you are later called to the clinic to see the doctor. You should hand this number to the nurses in the clinic when you are taken into the consulting room.

YOUR HISTORY will be taken by the doctor who will then decide which tests are required. You will normally be tested for the full range of sexually transmitted

---

Figure 3.1: Patient information leaflet

infections and a cervical smear will be taken if this has not been carried out recently, or if the doctor considers it important at the time of your examination. This is the one test which we consider important for your own GP to be aware of the result and to have recorded in your medical records. For this we will ask your consent to inform the GP and to forward the report to the surgery. If you do not wish this then you must return to the clinic to collect the report in 2–3 weeks. No cervical smear can be carried out without a contact address or telephone number for us to recall you should this be necessary.

The results of any tests carried out will be completed in approximately two weeks but some will be available before you leave the clinic and any treatment indicated will be given and discussed with you. Treatment is free and prescriptions are dispensed from the clinic.

A health adviser will be available to discuss the problems you have had and to help you avoid any difficulties in the future. She will advise you on the need for sexual partners, past and present, to be seen. This may be of concern to you, but it will be stressed that any details of partners which you disclose will be kept completely confidential and cannot be traced back to you.

FOLLOW-UP APPOINTMENTS It may be necessary to have regular treatment or for you to return to the clinic for further tests to ensure the infection has cleared. Please report to the GUM Reception Office before leaving to book your appointment. Every effort will be made to arrange treatments at times suitable to you to avoid the need for taking time off work should this be a problem to you, or a letter can be supplied for employers advising of the need for further appointments at the out patient department.

BLOOD TESTS As part of your full examination a blood test will be required. This is for sexually transmitted diseases and includes testing for hepatitis B but does not include a test for HIV. If you are worried and require testing for HIV please ask for an appointment for counselling at the time of booking in. It may be that this is the main requirement of attending the GUM clinic and appointments need not be booked for a full examination at the same visit. If HIV testing is required we must stress that the test and result are kept completely confidential and you must return to the clinic personally to be given the result.

RESULTS At no time will results be given to anyone other than yourself. For some results you may be asked to attend clinic or you may be asked to telephone for the results in two weeks' time, approximately when all are available.

FOLLOWING YOUR VISIT If you have any problems do not hesitate to contact the clinic again for advice. Before you leave you may have been advised on the need for salt/water washes following treatment or the need to drink water to relieve any discomfort when passing urine following the examination. If any such problems persist you may have to return for further treatment.

Figure 3.1: *Continued*
Taken from the Department of GUM information leaflet of East Glamorgan NHS Trust and reproduced with their kind permission.

the case of genital wart virus infection and the risks of recurrence; or the need to complete the full course of antibiotics and make a further appointment for repeat testing, to ensure a cure has been achieved. Patients should be warned of any complications that might arise during treatment, such as infection if adequate hygiene is not observed, for example in cases of wart virus or herpes virus infection.

The resumption of a normal sex life will be of concern and should be discussed. The advice given varies according to the condition, risks of re-infection by untreated partners and lifestyles of individuals. While in general advising no sex until treatment is complete, in some cases it may be more appropriate to stress the importance of condom use.

It can be important to raise the issues of fertility and pregnancy, possible risk to the neonate and methods of contraception in the future at a later stage of attendance at the GUM clinic, or the patient can be referred to family planning clinic.

It is also important to prepare the patient for the possibility of an unsuspected STD, including discussion about HIV infection, prior to results being available. Partner notification or contact tracing, as discussed in the first part of this chapter, should be carried out. It is important to give reasons for the need to see possibly asymptomatic partners, the consequences of partners not being treated and the risks of reinfection. Specific information, education and counselling on HIV infection should be offered and, where requested, pre-test counselling should be given and the need for post-test counselling stressed.

Risk reduction

'Information on its own is not enough to reduce the risk of STD transmission. The patient needs to be able to incorporate risk reduction into his or her life-style' (WHO, 1991). Specific information in relation to the different conditions will be found in the appropriate chapters of this book, but there are general principles in risk reduction practices that can be applied. The counsellor should be aware of the patient's lifestyle and give appropriate advice. Any changes made by the patient should not leave them isolated or separated from personal contact and the changes suggested should be achievable.

This will involve in-depth discussion about the patient's individual circumstances, lifestyle and relationships. Patients should be encouraged to consider the best solution to their own problems. How and when to raise the question of safer sex with partners and how to deal with possible risks where partners are uncooperative are important issues.

Patient education

Education may be defined as 'efforts aimed at producing positive changes in attitudes and in health and health-seeking behaviours in STDs and their prevention' (WHO, 1991).

How people learn can be considered under four basic principles:

1. Adults learn from one another as well as from the educator.
2. They learn from asking questions and getting answers. It is important to encourage this exchange.
3. Within a group setting, they learn from other people's questions and answers, especially the shy or inhibited. This may not be practical within the patient/professional relationship in the GUM clinic, but can be applied in the education of the young in school or young people's clinics, where the aim is the promotion of sexual health.
4. They learn from talking. By listening to the patient talk and encouraging them to disclose their fears, misinformation can be corrected and worries allayed.

The author's experience over many years has shown that patients want information. Some people have difficulty in remembering the advice and instructions they have been given by health professionals. One complaint that is repeatedly highlighted is the communication aspect. The principles of communication have been discussed in this chapter and it should be stressed that the best possible use should be made of the opportunities and time for patient education.

A busy clinic, where staff are pressurised, is not always the most appropriate place for patient education. A room where patients can be comfortable and where there will be no interruptions will facilitate the education process and should be available in all clinics.

Ewles and Simnett (1992) noted the main principles of patient education that can be used as a guide when giving information in relation to STDs. Important things should be said first. Key points need to be stressed and repeated to help patients remember them. It is important to give specific, precise advice and structure the information. Jargon should be avoided and simple language used. Appropriate use should be made of visual aids, leaflets and handouts. Care should be taken not to overload the patient with too much information and to give only relevant and realistic advice.

Health education literature, information on HIV, STDs and risk reduction should be on display in the patients' waiting area. Leaflets are available from the Health Education Authority and local health promotion departments and many drug companies produce appropriate patient education leaflets in relation to their products. Useful addresses of self-help groups and support groups are listed at the end of this chapter.

Videos can also be a useful source of information and if played in the patients' waiting area have been found to be beneficial as a teaching aid. Short video tapes can provide more information than posters or leaflets. They can also be used as a teaching method to raise awareness.

Television programmes are another useful aid to education. Most clinics report an increase in attenders on the days following a documentary on a specific infection, such as chlamydia. Also 'soaps', which are widely followed by young people, introduce specific topics into the storylines that raise public awareness. These can be used to open a discussion with patients, who can relate the programmes to their own symptoms.

Specific education on STDs must include the widely publicised principle of safer sex. This may mean different things to different people. Many young people have been exposed to this message through television, magazines and to a lesser extent, sex education within the school programme. They may be too embarrassed to confess that they have little knowledge of the correct way to use condoms, which is essential for maximum protection. Health educators should make sure that condom users understand and follow the instructions carefully. Even the well-educated may have difficulty following the instructions. Diagrams and a model can be used to demonstrate correct use and it should be emphasised that condom use is a skill that needs to be learned and practised. Patients may have never seen or touched a condom before and should be encouraged to do this and to practise putting on a condom, initially while alone, until confidence has been gained. Figure 3.2 gives practical advice on using a condom.

'Patients can be encouraged to view condom use as an enjoyable part of sex rather than as an unwelcome interruption. Where possible, information on condoms should be accompanied by free starter condoms. Patients should know where to obtain supplies' (WHO, 1991). It is particularly important to give information and education on condom use to newly sexually active young people. With the present knowledge and publicity surrounding the risks of unpro-

The following instructions on correct use should be discussed and demonstrated with an appropriate model or suitably shaped object:

1.   Use a new condom every time you have intercourse and don't use them after the expiry date on the packet. Condoms must be stored away from heat, light and moisture.
2.   Open the packet carefully to prevent the risk of tearing the condom. Care should be taken not to damage the condom with sharp nails or rings. Never use a damaged condom.
3.   Put the condom on as soon as the penis is erect but before any sexual contact has taken place.
4.   Squeeze the closed end of the condom to expel the air and to ensure it will unroll the correct way.
5.   Still squeezing the closed end, unroll gently down the full length of the penis.
6.   Only use a water based lubricant to prevent damage to the condom. A spermicidal lubricant would be suitable. Do not use saliva as a lubricant.
7.   If a condom tears during intercourse, withdraw the penis immediately and use a new condom.
8.   After making love, slowly withdraw the penis holding the condom in place at the base while the penis is still erect.
9.   Remove the condom carefully to prevent semen spillage and dispose of it after wrapping it in, for example, a tissue.

Figure 3.2: Use of condoms

tected sex, young people may be well informed of the possible exposure to HIV but less informed of the correct use of barrier methods of contraception, such as the condom. Information should be offered on the size, strength, flavour, colour and make of condom that is suitable for the culture and sexual orientation of the patient.

The GUM clinic may also offer contraceptive advice. In the future, where combined services may be offered, a full range of contraceptives should be available, rather than the present emphasis on condom use. However, when discussing exposure to STDs, patients may disclose a lack of adequate protection against unwanted pregnancy and the opportunity should be taken to discuss the various methods available and most suitable to the individual and their lifestyle. Post-coital contraception should be available and referral made to the family planning service where appropriate.

Many patients will have deep-seated fears surrounding STDs and the risks of HIV infection. Guilt following an extra-marital relationship, strict family background and upbringing, and shame where there has been a perceived promiscuous history may all lead to the need for ongoing counselling and psychiatric help. Referral to a psychologist, if not available within the service, may have to be made for those who are unable to deal with their problems and have presented at the clinic for help.

Other agencies that work closely with GUM services to provide holistic care and to which patients may require referral are shown in Table 3.3. Patients may also be referred to other departments within the NHS, such as psychiatric, X-ray, diabetic, dental and surgical, and also gynaecological or medical departments as appropriate.

Table 3.3: Outside agencies

* Social services
* Voluntary groups such as The Red Cross
* Housing agencies
* Community drug team
* British Pregnancy Advisory Service
* Rape Crisis

When a patient has been referred to a GUM clinic by their GP, the consultant will respond with information on the diagnosis and treatment given after attendance. If there has been self-referral, no such information is given without the patient's prior consent.

Focus groups

Certain patients presenting at a GUM clinic will require services specific to their individual needs. Knowledge of their lifestyles will be an essential part of understanding how these needs can be met.

Homosexuals/bisexuals/lesbians

Homosexuality in men and women, and attitudes to these groups, often has a strong cultural influence. When working in GUM, it is important to be non-judgmental with patients attending the clinic. A knowledge of human sexuality and variations of sexual behaviour, with the acceptance of those who do not appear to conform to the generally accepted societal 'norm', will encourage a greater degree of disclosure within the interview and enable fuller discussion in the promotion of sexual health. It is important to find out how the homosexual male has accepted his sexuality to be able to consider risk reducing activity as part of the education process. When there is an openness of their sexuality, a free discussion can be held, but a denial of orientation can lead to the need to address specific psycho-sexual problems and it may be more appropriate to refer to a specialist in this field. Male and female homosexuals may be considered within the following categories of behaviour determining their risk factor in sexual health:

1.   Two partners in a close relationship with sexual and personal satisfaction.
2.   Two partners living together but seeking extra sexual partners outside the relationship.
3.   Those who enjoy multiple sexual partners as part of their lifestyle.
4.   Those who have difficulty accepting their sexual orientation and in relating to others, particularly for sexual satisfaction.
5.   The 'loner' who has a poor self image and no involvement with other homosexuals.

The incidence of STDs is likely to be higher in males than females. This can be attributed to the difference in the choice of relationships within their orientation. 'It is a common misconception that male homosexuals invariably prefer effeminate male partners, and that homosexual women are attracted predominantly to other women possessing chiefly masculine traits. More often, the opposite is true, and like attracts like' (Beach, 1979).

On presentation at the GUM clinic, these patients will have the same anxieties as heterosexuals and the same issues will need to be addressed. In the homosexual male, fears of infection with HIV may be an important feature. The risk of hepatitis B infection should be discussed and immunisation offered, irrespective of the nature of diagnosis on attendance. Supplies of extra-strong condoms should be available to all homosexual men as part of the education in safer sex practices.

Drug users

In this group, those most at risk of infection from HIV, hepatitis B and hepatitis C are users who are injecting and who share needles. The partners of these attenders are also in a high-risk situation and both user and partner require counselling in relation to the possible exposure to blood-borne infection. Unfortunately, this group can also be the most difficult to follow up and tends to have a high default rate. With the patient's permission, referral to the Community Drug Team and Social Services may be required, if the patient is not already known to these agencies. When a patient is involved in injecting drug use, the habit is often funded either by crime or prostitution, and when crime is the means of obtaining the money to buy drugs, the inevitability of police involvement and prison can also be a factor in following up these cases.

Prostitution

As stated above, the need to fund a drug habit may lead to prostitution, either male or female, with all the attendant risks of multiple sexual partners. Regular health checks should be offered to all those involved in the sex industry. Many working girls are reluctant to attend but recognise the need to protect themselves, as sex is their livelihood and as such it is in their own interest to ensure they are regularly screened for STDs. In some areas, special centres are available where sex industry workers can have support and counselling along with full screening procedures, or encouragement is given to attend a GUM clinic.

Infertility

A brief mention of those who attend GUM clinics for investigation of infertility is important as a reminder of the complications that can occur if certain conditions, such as chlamydia infection, are not adequately treated at the time of diagnosis or where partners do not attend and re-infection occurs. Both males and females can be asymptomatic, so it is important to stress that all partners should be screened fully to ensure complications are minimised. The importance of giving health education and health promotion in relation to future fertility should be emphasised.

Erectile dysfunction

Over recent years there have been many changes in attitude, knowledge and treatment enabling more men to be treated for erectile dysfunction quickly, efficiently and at a reduced cost. This has led to GPs becoming more involved in what was previously a problem dealt with by a urologist or GUM clinic. However, these patients still require specialist skills in sexual counselling and a sound knowledge of the treatment options available and the medical conditions that can gradually lead to loss of libido and impotence. An important issue in the treatment is to 'consider the relationship of the patient and their partner as re-establishing erections after many years of sexual deprivation is usually associated with some trauma' (Hackett, 1995). Counselling of the partner should be part of the preliminary process, before the most appropriate form of treatment is offered.

Psychosexual counselling

'The provision by GUM clinics of treatment and advice in areas closely related to sexual health should be encouraged, given the necessary training and expertise among staff' (Allen & Hogg, 1993). The availability of a psychologist in a clinic can be an important contribution to the service in promotion of sexual health. Some patients attending with an STD may suffer an interruption to their sexual life only, but at worst considerable trauma may be experienced that will require long-term counselling and readjustment. Fear of exposure to HIV or of possible pregnancy, particularly where this follows an extra-marital relationship, can produce long-term psychological effects on the regular relationship.

Non-consummation of a relationship may also be referred to a GUM clinic for examination to rule out physical causes. Psychosexual counselling can do a great deal to help couples with their problems when no physical cause has been identified. This is time consuming within a busy clinic setting, but rewarding when patients are satisfied following successful counselling.

Stress in modern life and attendant complications within relationships allow those working in the field of GUM the opportunity to extend and expand services to patients and can only benefit the service as a whole.

The following range of services are offered within the author's GUM clinic at Pontypridd:

- well woman/well man
- screening for STDs
- cytology – screening and counselling
- gynaecological problems and referrals
- colposcopy – screening, counselling and treatment following abnormal cytology result
- management, care and treatment of HIV positive patients
- counselling services for the worried well
- contact tracing
- psychosexual counselling and treatment or referral
- health education and health promotion
- family planning advice
- post-coital information and treatment
- pregnancy testing.

Counselling services are provided with all of the above and domiciliary visits are offered for all the services. Advice and service is not only offered to the patients, but also to partners and relatives.

Not all clinics will be able to offer this range of services, but they will be able to access such services as required. A list of contact names and addresses for further information and/or support for patients is included at the end of this chapter.

The aims of the author's clinic are outlined in Figure 3.3.

O — Our **O**bjective is to treat patients as individuals and to encourage aware-ness of a healthier lifestyle

P — Our **P**atient care and clinical practice will be responsive to the changing needs of society

D — Our **D**esire is to create a friendly and safe environment

G — Our **G**oal can only be met by

U — The client helping **U**s to **U**nderstand your needs and by all staff being

M — **M**otivated to fulfil those needs and the standards we have set for our department

---

Figure 3.3: Aims of the out patient department

Conclusion

Until further research proves otherwise, education is going to continue to be the main weapon against the spread of STDs, includ-ing HIV. It will remain the principal aim of those working in GUM to provide open and readily available access for anyone seeking a healthier sexual lifestyle.

Acknowledgement

The author would like to acknowledge the help and support she received from her previous manager, Colleen Thomas (Senior Nurse Manager, Department of GU Medicine, Pontypridd), now retired.

References

Adler MW (1990) ABC of Sexually Transmitted Diseases, 2nd edn. London: British Medical Association.

Allen I, Hogg D (1993) Work Roles and Responsibilities in Genitourinary Medicine Clinics. London: Policy Studies Institute.

Beach FA (1979) Animal models for human sexuality. In: CIBA Foundation Symposium. 62:113–43.

British Medical Association, General Medical Services Committee, Health Education Authority, Brook Advisory Centres, Family Planning Association, Royal College of General Practitioners (undated) Confidentiality and People under 16. London: British Medical Association.

Craig DG (1990) Medicolegal problems in rape in the United Kingdom. In: Csonka GW & Oates JK (Eds) Sexuality Transmitted Diseases – A Textbook of Genitourinary Medicine. London: Baillière Tindall.

DOH (1993) The Health of the Nation: Key Area Handbook HIV/AIDS & Sexual Health. London: HMSO.

Evans BA (1990) Introduction. In: Csonka GW & Oates JK (Eds) Sexually Transmitted Diseases – A Textbook of Genitourinary Medicine. London: Baillière Tindall.

Ewles L, Simnett I (1992) Promoting Health: A Practical Guide, 2nd edn. London: Scutari Press.

Hackett G (1995) The general practice management of erectile dysfunction. The Journal of Sexual Health (March/April): 9–11.

Miller R, Bor R (1989) AIDS A Guide to Clinical Counselling. London: Scutari Press.

Nelson-Jones R (1986) Human Relationship Skills Training and Self-help. London: Cassell Educational Ltd.

Robertson DHH, McMillan A, Young H (1989) Clinical Practice in Sexually Transmissible Diseases, 2nd edn. Edinburgh: Churchill Livingstone.

Stedman Y, Elstein M (1995) Rethinking sexual health clinics. British Medical Journal 310 (February): 342–3.

World Health Organization (1991) Management of Patients with Sexually Transmitted Diseases. Geneva: WHO.

Bibliography

Adler M, Johnson A (1993) British Journal of Hospital Medicine and Sexual Health: HIV/AIDS 49. Royal Society of Medical Press.

Blakely V (1993) Conference Report: Public Education on Sexually Transmitted Diseases. Health Promotion Wales.

Guillebaud J (1991) The Pill. Oxford: University Press

Holmes KK, Mårdh P-A, Sparling PF, Weisner PJ (Eds) (1990) Sexually Transmitted Diseases, 2nd edn. New York: McGraw-Hill.

Jones K, Tilford S (1994) Health Education: Effectiveness, Efficiency & Equity, 2nd edn. London: Chapman & Hall.

UKCC (1991) Exercising Accountability. London: UKCC.

UKCC (1992) Code of Professional Conduct. London: UKCC.

UKCC (1992) The Scope of Professional Practice. London: UKCC.

Helplines and support groups

Acceptance, 64 Holmside Avenue, Sheerness, Kent HE12 3EY. Tel: 01795 661463
(Tues–Fri 7pm–9pm)
Helpline/support group for parents of lesbians and gay men.

AIDS Ahead, The Facts Centre, 23–25 Weston Park, London N8 9SY.
Albert Kennedy Trust. Tel: 0161 953 4059
For homeless lesbian and gay teenagers.

Association of Community Health Councils for England & Wales, 30 Drayton Park, London N5 1PB. Tel: 0171 609 8405
The Association set up by the NHS (Association of Community Health Councils) Regulations 1977 under the 1973 Act to advise and help councils in the performance of their functions and to represent at the national level the consumer interest in the health service.

AVERT. Tel: 01403 210202
For booklets, information and research reports on HIV and AIDS.

BEDS, British Erectile Dysfunction Society
Enquiries to Dr W.W. Dinsmore, The Royal Society of Medicine, 1 Wimpole Street, London. W1M 7AA

Body Positive, 51B Philbeach Gardens, Earls Court, London SW5 9EB, Tel: 0171 373 9124
Offers support and advice for people who are HIV/HTLV-3 antibody positive. Telephone counselling service run by volunteers, face to face and group counselling. Social and health promotion activities hospital visiting.

British Association for Counselling, 37a Sheep Street, Rugby, Warwickshire CV21 3BX. Tel: 01788 78328
Represents counsellors in the British Isles, provides information to the public on where counselling is available nationally.

British Herbal Medicine Association, PO Box 304, Bournemouth BH7 6JX. Tel: 01202 433691
Exists to defend the right of the public to use herbal remedies and to have free access to them, encourages wider knowledge and recognition of herbal remedies by medical practitioners, promotes high standards of quality and safety in herbal remedies.

British Homeopathic Association, 27a Devonshire Street, London W1N 1RJ. Tel: 0171 935 2163
Works to extend the knowledge and use of homeopathy amongst people in all walks of life.

British Hypnotherapy Association, 1 Wytburn Place, London W1H 5WL. Tel: 0171 723 4443
Professional organisation that maintains a register of qualified practitioners trained to resolve emotional or behavioural problems through psychotherapy and when relevant, hypnosis.

British Pregnancy Advisory Service (BPAS), 7 Belgrave Road, London SW1V 1QB. Tel: 0171 828 2484
Carries out pregnancy tests, abortions, vasectomy, sterilisation and infertility investigations and referrals.

Brook Advisory Centres (Head Office), 153a East Street, London SE17 2SD. Tel: 0171 708 1234
Has 21 centres providing free and confidential service offering contraceptive advice and supplies, pregnancy testing, abortion referral, pregnancy counselling, and counselling for sexual and emotional problems.

Community Health Group for Ethnic Minorities, 2nd Floor, 13 Macclesfield Street, London W1V 7HL. Tel: 0171 740 6155 Answerphone
Provides free 24-hour interpreting and translating service for health care and social workers in over 20 languages. Also offers information service and a comprehensive reference library in the field of health and race.

Cytomegalovirus Support Group, 69 The Leasowes, Ford, Shrewsbury, Shropshire SY5 9LU. Tel: 01743 850055
Support group for parents with children with congenital cytomegalovirus.

Family Planning Association, 27–35 Mortimer Street, London W1N 7RJ. Tel: 0171 636 7866
Runs an education unit and produces literature on family planning.

FFLAG (Families and Friends of Lesbians & Gays), PO Box 153, Manchester M60 1LP. Tel: 0161 748 3452
For your local helpline / support group.

Friend. Tel: 0171 837 3337
(Daily 7.30pm–10.00pm)
A befriending and counselling service with many local groups.

Gay Bereavement Project, The Unitarian Rooms, Hoop Lane, London NW11 8BS. Tel: 0181 455 8894.

Gay Men Fighting AIDS. Tel: 0171 738 6872
For information on safer sex for gay men.

Gay Times. By subscription to: Subscription Department (1955), Mellivres Ltd, Worldwide House, 116–134 Bayham Street, London NW1 0BA – or from newsagents
Magazine with up-to-date information on gay issues and detailed listings of local clubs / pubs / meeting places and support groups.

The Haemophilia Society, PO Box 9, 16 Trinity Street, London SE1 1DE. Tel: 0171 407 1010.

The Health Education Authority, Hamilton House, Mabledon Place, London WC1H 9TX. Tel: 0171 383 3933
For information leaflets, posters and education lists for teaching sessions – local number in telephone directory.

Lesbian & Gay Switchboard, BM Switchboard, London WC1N 3XX. Tel: 0171 837 7324 (24 hrs)
Advice and information on local support groups.

London Rape Crisis Centre, P.O. Box 69, London WC1X 9NJ. Tel: 0171 916 5466 (Office 9am–5pm) 0171 837 1600 (Counselling line 10am–10pm).

Mainliners, P.O. Box 125, London SW9 8EF. Tel: 0171 737 3141
Advice for drug users and ex-drug users who have concerns about HIV/AIDS.

MESMAC (for Deaf), BDA Health Promotion Services, 17 Macon Court, Herald
Drive, Crewe, Cheshire CW1 1EA. Tel: 0181 341 4848. Voice line: 01270 250
736.

National AIDS Helpline. Tel: 0800 567 123 FREE-24 hrs.

Positively Women, 5 Sebastian Street, London EC1V 0HE. Tel: 0171 490 5515
Offers support and counselling to women with HIV.

The Praed Street Project, The Jefferis Wing Centre for Sexual Health, St Mary's
Hospital, Paddington, London W2 1NY. Tel: 0171 725 6619
A free and confidential specialist sexual health service for women working in the sex industry.

Pregnancy Advisory Service, 11–13 Charlotte Street, London W1P 1HD. Tel:
0171 637 8962
*Performs terminations, pregnancy testing, AID, morning after contraception, cervical smears, coun-
selling (pregnancy and post abortion), vasectomies and sterilisations.*

REGARD (National Disabled Lesbian and Gay Organisations), BM Regard,
London,WC1N 3XX.

Relate (formerly The Marriage Guidance Council), Herbert Grey College, Little
Church Street, Rugby, Warwickshire CV21 3AP. Tel: 01788 573241.

SHAKTI (South Asian Lesbian and Gay Network). Tel: 0171 278 7856.

The Terrence Higgins Trust, BM AIDS, London WC1 3XX. Tel: 0171 242 1010
(Helpline) – 0171 831 0330 (administration).
Offers information, advice and support regarding HIV/AIDS

Womens Aid Federation (England) Ltd, PO Box 391, Bristol BS99 7WS. Tel: 0117
963 3542
*National office for women's groups that provide temporary refuge accommodation, advice and
support to women and their children who are suffering physical, mental or sexual abuse.*

Chapter 4
Syphilis

Malcolm Gowardun

Introduction

Syphilis is one of the most interesting sexually transmitted diseases (STDs) worldwide. In the UK, it is far less common than other STDs, but it is still important because if left untreated it is chronic and potentially fatal. It may also be passed on during pregnancy to the unborn child (congenital syphilis).

The causative organism of syphilis is *Treponema pallidum*, 'the pale twisted thread' (Oates, 1969), which belongs to the family *Treponematoceae*. It was formerly known as *Spirochaeta pallidum*. Other types of treponema that can infect humans are *T. pertenue* (yaws), *T. endemicum* (bejel) and *T. carateum* (pinta). A treponeme of low pathogenicity, which may be found in the male genital area, is *T. balanitidis* and there have been non-pathogenic treponemes isolated from the mouth (Csonka & Oates, 1990; Tramont, 1990).

T. pallidum is a motile, corkscrew-shaped organism made up of six to 18 coils, evenly disposed, and it replicates about once every 30–32 hours (Csonka & Oates, 1990). It is easily killed by drying and sunlight (Oates, 1969). Culture in the laboratory has not been successful, making studies of the organism very limited (Musher, 1990). Three movements appear to propel the organism: slow undulation, corkscrew-like rotation and sluggish backward and forward motion. It also tends to bend at right angles (jack knifes) in the middle.

Even though small amounts of treponemes can cause infection, they die rapidly once outside the body. The risk of acquiring syphilis through sexual exposure with a person who has active syphilis in a lesion on the skin or mucous membrane is said to be up to 60%

(Thin, 1990). Csonka and Oates (1990) put this figure nearer to 20–25% following a single exposure. Late stage syphilis is not infectious.

Transmission and incubation period

Most cases of syphilis are acquired by sexual contact (Robertson, McMillan & Young, 1989), with the exception of congenital syphilis, where it is possible for the foetus to acquire it *in utero* from a syphilitic mother (Chang et al., 1995). Asexual transmission of syphilis is possible through kissing or touching a person with active lesions, transfusion of infected blood or accidental inoculation, for example needlestick injury (Tramont, 1990). Transmission of syphilis through blood transfusion is rare in the developed world today, due to low incidence of the disease and screening of blood donors. But more importantly, Robertson, McMillan and Young (1989) note that fresh blood is rarely used these days and treponemes do not survive after being stored at −10 °C to −20 °C for more than a few days.

Treponemes can enter the body through small abrasions in the skin and can also penetrate unbroken mucous membrane. They make their way to the local lymphatic glands, usually the inguinal glands, and soon enter the bloodstream where they are carried to the other tissues of the body. Factors such as sexual behaviour, hygiene, immune status and inoculum size also affect the risk of transmission (Tramont, 1990). On average, the incubation period for this infection is around 25 days, though it may range from 9–90 days (Robertson, McMillan & Young, 1989).

History

When researching syphilis, one cannot fail to learn something of its history. Syphilis received its name from a poem written by Fracastoro about an infected shepherd named Syphilus (Sparling, 1990). References to this venereal disease in the Bible indicate that it existed in the Middle East and therefore probably in Europe, prior to the birth of Christ, while some scholars suggest that it has only existed in Europe since the voyages of Christopher Columbus in the late fifteenth century (Caffyn-Parsons, 1978). A third theory, described by Hudson in 1946 as the Unitarian theory, is that all treponemal infections are caused by one organism, namely *T. pallidum*, which originated in sub-Saharan Africa (Waugh, 1991).

In the late fifteenth century, people from every European country joined with King Charles VIII of France to besiege Naples, but they became afflicted with the pox from women spreading syphilis to friends and foe alike. This new disease, the Great Pox (as distinguished from smallpox), then spread throughout Europe, reaching Paris, Geneva, Nuremberg and Bristol in 1496, Aberdeen and Edinburgh by 1497 and Russia by 1499 (Waugh, 1991). Evans (1994) describes how by the late eighteenth century, when the incidence of syphilis was at its peak, it had nearly 400 names such as 'German Pox', 'French Pox' and 'Portuguese Disease', each country blaming another for its origin.

It was in the eighteenth century that syphilis was recognised as a sexually transmitted infection. Prior to this, it had not been appreciated as such and it was not until much later that the chronic nature of the disease was recognised (Csonka & Oates, 1990). Gonorrhoea and syphilis were believed to be one and the same infection until the difference was established in 1838 by the French physician Philippe Ricord. The major advances that have followed this century, noted by Csonka and Oates (1990) and Thin (1990), are shown in Table 4.1.

Table 4.1: Syphilis: advances this century

1903	Primates successfully inoculated with syphilis: **Metchnikoff & Rowe**
1905	*T. pallidum* discovered: **Schaudinn & Hoffman**
1906	*T. pallidum* demonstrated using dark-field microscopy: **Landsteiner**
1906	Development of first serological test for syphilis: **Wassermann**
1910	Discovery of salvarsan, the first effective drug against syphilis: **Enrlich & Hata**
1917	Malarial therapy used as treatment of neurosyphilis (halving the mortality of general paresis): **Wagner-Jauregg**
1928	Discovery of penicillin, used as treatment for syphilis since 1943 which changed the prognosis of the disease: **Fleming**
1946	Development of Venereal Disease Research Laboratory (VDRL) test: **Harris**
1949	Development of *T. pallidum* immobilisation (TPI) test, the first specific reaction in the diagnosis of syphilis: **Nelson & Mayer**

Incidence

Some form of syphilis may always have been present. Descriptions over the centuries make it clear that it has always been a severe contagious disease that was often fatal (Csonka & Oates, 1990). The disease pattern is now milder, especially in neurosyphilis, although it is unclear if this is due to changes in the organism or the gradual development of some immunity.

Waugh (1991) reports that in times of war, a rise in the number of cases of venereal disease has been observed. He also states that syphilis had a tremendous impact on the two World Wars and became the subject of the Final Report of the Royal Commission on Venereal Disease in 1916, the principles of which are still important today.

Syphilis is more prevalent in men than women and evidence of cardiovascular and neurological syphilis is more common in men (Csonka & Oates, 1990). Primarily, the disease affects young people between 20 and 35 years of age (Benenson, 1990).

The incidence of syphilis in the UK is shown in Figure 4.1. It has fallen dramatically since 1945, post Second World War (Thin, 1990). Csonka and Oates (1990) attribute this to the introduction of penicillin, which led experts of the early 1950s to believe that syphilis would soon be controlled if not eliminated, though they note that cases increased worldwide as oral contraceptives were used and heterosexual and homosexual promiscuity increased.

Until the mid-1980s and the advent of acquired immune deficiency syndrome (AIDS), when safer sex practices were more widely adopted, the incidence of syphilis reported in homosexual men was high (Tramont, 1990). Syphilis remains a problem in developing countries and is a current problem in the USA (Goldmeier & Hay,

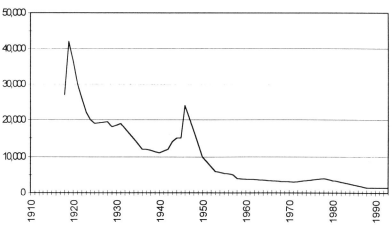

Number of new cases

Figure 4.1: Incidence of syphilis 1918–1994 in the UK

1993). In the late 1980s and early 1990s, there was an increase in syphilis despite human immunodeficiency virus (HIV) and syphilis prevention programmes being in place (St Louis, Farley & Aral, 1996). In the south-eastern United States, factors such as poverty, minority race and ethnicity, and geographic clustering appear to contribute to the persistent syphilis morbidity (Aral, 1996).

Linglöf (1995) reports that the incidence of syphilis has risen in Russia and the Baltic States since 1991, when they regained their independence. He suggests that the factors causing this rise may be due to increased travel across open borders, adoption of western lifestyle and a more accessible sex industry with increased prostitution.

In the United Kingdom, a decrease of 4% in new cases of syphilis was reported between 1991 and 1992. The number of all new cases in 1994 was 1393, of which there were 304 new cases of infectious syphilis, a fall of 10% over the previous year, with males accounting for 64% of new infection. The total of 1393 cases is the lowest recorded since the late 1980s (DOH, 1995).

Classification

In an attempt to describe the clinical process of syphilis in the human body, it is usual to divide it into the acquired form and the congenital form. The acquired form of the disease is commonly divided into three stages: early infectious or primary and secondary; latent which is subdivided into early latent and late latent; and tertiary or late syphilis. Congenital syphilis is divided into early congenital aged up to 2 years and late congenital over 2 years (Robertson, McMillan & Young, 1989).

The primary stage refers to the incubation period and the development of a primary lesion at the site of inoculation, known as a chancre (Adler, 1990). Secondary syphilis usually occurs 6 to 8 weeks after the appearance of the chancre, with about one third of patients still having the primary lesion present (Robertson, McMillan & Young, 1989). In secondary syphilis, lesions may affect the skin and mucous membranes anywhere on the body.

Csonka and Oates (1990) describe the subdivisions of latent syphilis as early (less than 2 years' duration) and late (more than 2 years' duration). During the latent phase, the patient is asymptomatic though they have never been treated.

Late syphilis, otherwise known as tertiary syphilis, may present 3 to 20 years after exposure but is rarely seen in this country nowadays

(Adler, 1990). It takes the form of neurosyphilis, cardiovascular syphilis or gummatous syphilis.

Primary syphilis

When the spirochaete has penetrated its new host, it begins to multiply at the site of its entrance and during the next 10–90 days a primary sore appears, which is usually on the genitalia (Csonka & Oates, 1990). The chancre is usually solitary, painless and may go unnoticed (Adler, 1990), though patients infected with HIV may have multiple chancres (Tramont, 1990). The lesion presents as a red spot, which progresses to a round ulcer with an indurated base and edges (Adler, 1990).

In heterosexual men, the common sites for a primary lesion are the coronal sulcus, the glans penis, the inner surface of the preputial sac, the frenum and the urinary meatus, although the shaft of the penis and extragenital areas may also be affected. In homosexual men, the chancre often presents in the anal canal and can be mistaken for an anal fissure. In women, the vulva and the labia are commonly affected and, rarely, the cervix. Less commonly in either sex, the lesion may appear on the lips, tonsils, fingers, buttocks or nipples (Csonka & Oates, 1990). Local lymphadenopathy may accompany the lesion, usually bilaterally, nodes being firm, freely mobile and painless.

Secondary syphilis

T. pallidum disseminates quickly throughout the body via the circulatory system and signs of secondary syphilis can be observed 3 to 6 weeks after the primary chancre appears (Thin, 1990). The manifestations of secondary syphilis can include skin lesions, genital lesions, lesions in the mouth and throat, constitutional symptoms, central nervous system (CNS) symptoms, and eye, ear, renal and gastrointestinal symptoms.

Secondary syphilis lesions can be very variable and widespread and are seen in over 80% of patients with syphilis (Robertson, McMillan & Young, 1989). The so-called secondary rash is characteristically a generalised non-irritating rash, pale red in colour. The rash remains for several weeks, does not ulcerate and is often associated with symptoms such as malaise, slight fever and generalised enlargement of the glands. Csonka and Oates (1990) describe the rash as commonly being macular, but it may be papular and slightly scaly. With time the rash becomes much less noticeable and may appear greyish on dark skin.

The distribution of the rash helps to diagnose the condition, as characteristically, it covers the trunk, arms and legs, but also it can be especially prominent on the face, the palms of the hands and the soles of the feet (Csonka & Oates, 1990). In warm, moist regions of the body, such as the perineum, skin lesions may proliferate into large, fleshy wart-like lesions known as 'condylomata lata', which are highly infectious and contain vast numbers of treponemes (Robertson, McMillan & Young, 1989).

'Snail-track ulcers' are another feature of secondary syphilis, relating to irregular greyish patches on the mucous membranes covering the oro-pharynx, naso-pharynx, larynx and male and female genitalia (Adler, 1990). If the lips and oro-pharynx are affected in this way, this is when 'the treponema can be transmitted to other individuals by kissing, or rarely, by means of other objects such as a shared drinking vessel' (Oates, 1969).

Csonka and Oates (1990) report that some people have problems with photophobia, severe nocturnal headaches and neck stiffness, due to involvement of the meninges. Analysis of the cerebrospinal fluid (CSF) reveals an increase in the number of white blood cells (pleocytosis) and total protein, consistent with this meningeal picture. Mild constitutional symptoms are often present, for example malaise, muscular and bone pain and a sore throat (Csonka & Oates, 1990). Also, hair loss may occur and it is usually patchy, giving the scalp a 'moth-eaten' appearance (Robertson, McMillan & Young, 1989). When the rash has subsided, the patient appears asymptomatic and enters the early latent stage of the disease (Zenker & Rolfs, 1990) but is still able to transmit the disease during relapses of secondary syphilis.

Diagnosis of primary syphilis

Thin (1990) describes the first factor to aid diagnosis of primary syphilis as being clinical suspicion, bearing in mind the age of the patient, their sexual behaviour and contact history. Also, a solitary, indurated, non-tender ulcer may be suggestive of primary syphilis, whereas multiple painful lesions reduce the probability and differentiation must be made to exclude other causes such as genital herpes, trauma, fixed drug eruption, etc.

Dark-field microscopy

Dark-field microscopy is usually the first investigation performed to confirm a diagnosis of syphilis. It may be the only way to establish a positive diagnosis in the first instance, as serological tests do not give positive results in primary syphilis until about 2 weeks after the chancre presents (Adler, 1990). In order to obtain a good specimen for examination, the surface of the lesion must be cleaned thoroughly with gauze soaked in physiological saline and it is important to squeeze the lesion and scrape it firmly to collect serum rather than blood (Thin, 1990). The serous exudate is then placed on to two or three glass slides, depending on clinic policy. A drop of saline may be added to the slides, as described in Chapter 1. After a coverslip has been placed on the material it is ready for dark-field microscopy using the oil-immersion objective. Thin (1990) states that *T. pallidum* can be readily identified by an experienced microscopist from its characteristic features and movements.

Researchers stress that if the initial dark-field microscopy examination is negative in a suspected case, the procedure should be repeated on at least two successive days (Thin, 1990). The patient may be advised to bathe the lesion with normal saline between examinations, to reduce the risk of secondary infection. A negative result does not exclude syphilis, as it may be that the lesion is healing or there are just too few organisms to be identified. Thin (1990) also goes on to point out that topical or systemic treatment may have already been given and that secondary infection may obscure the field.

Serological tests

Venepuncture is a common procedure carried out by nurses in genito-urinary medicine (GUM) clinics to obtain blood samples for serological screening, a routine investigation for most patients during the course of their attendance. Serological testing for syphilis may be described as a diagnostic test, applied to patients with signs and symptoms of the disease, or as a screening test, applied to patients in the absence of any clinical manifestations (Schmid, 1996). The practice of screening for syphilis during pregnancy, using serological tests, is well established in British antenatal clinics to prevent congenital syphilis (Boot et al., 1992). Serological tests are divided into non-specific and specific, according to the antibodies they detect.

Tests to detect non-specific treponemal antibodies:

Venereal Disease Research Laboratory (VDRL) test

The VDRL test is the standard test for routine screening for syphilis. It is simple, quick and cheap to perform and depends on the ability of heated serum to flocculate, i.e. produce visible antigen–antibody complexes when mixed with cardiolipin-cholesterol-lecithin antigen (Robertson, McMillan & Young, 1989). The test will only give positive results in up to 75% of cases of primary syphilis, as seroconversion takes 3 to 5 weeks after contracting the infection (Adler, 1990). Seroconversion may take longer in patients infected with HIV (Goldmeier & Hay, 1993) and it is known that the patient's blood test may always be negative if primary syphilis is treated before seroconversion takes place (Csonka & Oates, 1990). It is important to remember that a diagnosis of syphilis should not be made on the basis of one positive VDRL test result, as other treponemal conditions, for example yaws, give rise to positive results. Error in laboratory handling and testing (El-Zaatari & Martens, 1994) and also biological false positive (BFP) reactions are possible (Adler, 1990), which may be acute or chronic. Acute BFP reactions have been reported in pregnancy, drug addiction, after acute viral infections and in healthy people and only last up to 6 months (Smikle, James & Prabhakar, 1990). Chronic BFP reactions last indefinitely and are seen more particularly in auto-immune diseases, for example systemic lupus erythematosus (SLE) and rheumatoid arthritis (Adler, 1990). When BFP reactions are seen, specific tests for syphilis will be negative.

The VDRL test is a useful indicator to assess disease activity and the patient's response to treatment (Tramont, 1990). The antigen titre should decrease following treatment of primary or early secondary syphilis, reaching seronegativity within a year, but if treatment is delayed a low lipoidal antigen titre may persist (Csonka & Oates, 1990).

Rapid plasma reagin (RPR) test

This is an adaptation of the VDRL test. Robertson, McMillan and Young (1989) describe how the VDRL test antigen, after being suspended in choline chloride and having a chelating agent added, can remain stable for up to 6 months when stored at 4–10 °C. They also say that with the addition of finely separated carbon particles to the antigen, test results can be observed with the naked eye. Though it is a more expensive test to produce than the simple VDRL test, it is valuable in blood banks and laboratories (Tramont, 1990) and in field studies in developing countries (Robertson, McMillan & Young, 1989). It is often referred to as the RPR card test, as the antigen is marked in circles on plastic cards.

Automated reagin test

This is similar to the RPR test but uses auto-analyser equipment and is more especially useful in blood transfusion centre laboratories (Robertson, McMillan & Young, 1989).

Wassermann reaction (WR)

This was the first serological test for syphilis, introduced by Wassermann in 1906. It has now been discontinued and superseded by the VDRL and reagin tests.

Tests to detect specific antitreponemal antibodies:

Smikle, James and Prabhakar (1990) recommend that 'confirmatory tests should be performed on all sera with a positive VDRL'. These specific tests have developed from the original *T. pallidum* immobilisation (TPI) test, developed by Nelson and Mayer in 1949 (Csonka & Oates, 1990).

T. pallidum haemagglutination (TPHA) test

Adler (1990) and Csonka and Oates (1990) agree that the combination of VDRL and TPHA tests is the simplest and best method of routine screening for treponemal disease.

The TPHA test is the last of the serological tests to become positive but is very specific. It will be positive in only 60% of patients with primary syphilis but it will always be positive in the secondary stages (Adler, 1990). False positive results can occur in up to 2% of samples (Csonka & Oates, 1990).

Fluorescent treponemal antibody absorbed (FTA-ABS) test

This test is the first of the serological tests to become positive. Although it is not a suitable test for routine screening, it is a confirmatory test widely used when any of the routine screening tests are positive (Tramont, 1990). In patients with primary syphilis, the test is positive in 85–90% of cases (Adler, 1990). Invariably, this test continues to be positive for life, irrespective of whether treatment for syphilis is given.

The patient's serum is first treated with a non-pathogenic treponemal antigen or 'sorbent', to remove cross-reacting antibodies. The specific antigen for this test is derived from *T. pallidum* harvested from rabbit testes. By use of the indirect immunofluorescence technique, specific serum antibodies are demonstrated by bright apple-green fluorescence of the treponemes (Robertson, McMillan & Young, 1989).

Diagnosis of secondary syphilis

Dark-field microscopy

Dark-field microscopy should always be undertaken on serum from papules, condylomata lata or a mucous patch (Thin, 1990). However, in mouth lesions the ubiquitous presence of non-pathogenic treponemes often causes confusion.

Serological tests

Serological tests for secondary syphilis are the most dependable, as they are always positive and the reagin (either RPR card test or the VDRL) reaction shows a high and rising titre at this stage of the disease. Thin (1990) suggests that clinical manifestations, repeated reactive results to the RPR card test or VDRL test in titre 1:16 or higher and a positive FTA-ABS result confirm a presumptive diagnosis of secondary syphilis. A skin biopsy may also be helpful but is not often required.

Treatment of early acquired syphilis (primary and secondary)

Neoarsphenamine and bismuth were used to treat nearly all syphilis in the pre-penicillin era, though with severe side effects. Intramuscular penicillin as a treatment for syphilis was regarded as a miracle drug when it was first introduced. Although penicillin is an extremely successful treatment for syphilis, the optimal dose is still not known (Zenker & Rolfs, 1990) as there is a paucity of good scientific data available (Goldmeier & Hay, 1993). However, it is the drug of choice in the UK today, and the aim is to maintain a prolonged low concentration of penicillin in the blood. Procaine penicillin is more suitable than other penicillin preparations (Csonka & Oates, 1990), though treatment regimens vary from clinic to clinic. Csonka and Oates also note that the World Health Organization (WHO) recommends that procaine penicillin 600 000 IU (600 mg) daily is given for 10 to 20 days, depending on the stage of the disease. The GUM nurse must emphasise to the patient that this course of injections must be completed to ensure a cure. If the patient fails to attend daily, the course of injections has to be restarted.

It is usual to arrange for the Accident and Emergency department staff to administer the injections at the weekend. Alternatively, a more compliant regimen is benzathine penicillin 2.4 mega units intramuscularly, weekly for three consecutive weeks. This option is not advocated by Csonka and Oates (1990) as it does not produce treponemicidal levels within the CSF, which potentially gives rise to neurosyphilis, and it has been noted that when treating patients also infected with HIV, 'higher and prolonged doses of penicillin should be considered' (Savall, Valls & Cabre, 1991). For developing countries, Goeman et al. (1995) are of the opinion that benzathine penicillin is still the easiest treatment.

Patients receiving a course of daily injections may be working and may therefore need to make special arrangements to attend for treatment. These patients will need constant support by the nursing staff and should be reassured that they will be cured. The daily injection can be painful, so it is important to administer the injections in alternate buttocks. Most patients who receive benzathine penicillin experience excruciating pain during and following the injections. It may, therefore, be advisable for them to take a mild painkiller, such as paracetamol 1 g, just before the injection. Moreover, patients may find it soothing to sit in a warm bath and rub their buttocks well with a towel.

Alternatives to penicillin

If a patient is allergic to penicillin or is unable to attend daily for injections, then tetracycline 500 mg may be given orally four times a day, for 15 days to treat early syphilis or 30 days to treat latent syphilis (Csonka & Oates, 1990).

Other regimens, such as erythromycin or oxytetracycline 500 mg orally four times a day for 30 days, may be prescribed (Adler, 1990). Chloramphenicol, ceftriaxone and other cephalosporins have all proved to be effective treatments for early syphilis (Tramont, 1990). As the cure rate with these alternatives is less successful than penicillin, Adler (1990) notes that some doctors will repeat treatment after 3 months. Relapse after adequate treatment with penicillin is very rare (Robertson, McMillan & Young, 1989).

Side effects of treatment

Jarisch-Herxheimer reaction (JHR)

It is well documented that the Jarisch-Herxheimer reaction (JHR) occurs in many patients within a short time of receiving treatment for syphilis, especially penicillin (Zenker & Rolfs, 1990; Goldmeier & Hay, 1993).

This acute, transient, systemic inflammatory reaction was first described in 1895 by Jarisch, and confirmed in 1902 by Herxheimer and Krause, as an exacerbation in the appearance of skin lesions in early syphilis after initiating treatment with mercury (Robertson, McMillan & Young, 1989). The most common reaction is mild and consists of flu-like symptoms and exacerbation of skin lesions (Goldmeier & Hay, 1993). The event occurs 3 to 12 hours following the first injection (Adler, 1990) and lasts 12 to 24 hours (Zenker & Rolfs, 1990). The reaction is most common with treatment of secondary syphilis, but may be seen in any stage (Tramont, 1990). The incidence of JHR reported by Csonka and Oates (1990) is shown in Table 4.2.

Table 4.2: Incidence of Jarisch-Herxheimer reaction

Primary	50%
Secondary	90%
Early latent	25%
Late (tertiary)	Rare

The mechanism of Jarisch-Herxheimer reaction is not fully understood, but the patient can be reassured that the reaction will not happen with further treatment (Csonka & Oates, 1990). In early syphilis the reaction is harmless, but before administering the first treatment the nurse must advise the patient to expect a mild febrile reaction. Rest, fluids and aspirin or paracetamol tablets are the treatment advised (Thin, 1990). In late syphilis, the reaction can be much more serious and the patient's condition should be monitored closely following initial treatment (Goldmeier & Hay, 1993). Systemic steroids may reduce peak temperatures.

Procaine penicillin reaction

Nurses should be aware of two significant reactions to procaine penicillin, described by Csonka and Oates (1990) as:

1. The patient feeling as though they are dying, being very worried and feeling depersonalised. In some cases, the patient becomes hysterical, before the reaction passes off spontaneously.
2. A reaction is similar to the above but accompanied by hypertension, tachycardia, hyperventilation and vomiting. On occasions, cardiovascular collapse has been reported but there have not been any fatalities recorded.

Follow-up after treatment

According to Thin (1990), treatment failure has been reported for early syphilis in up to 10% of cases and he believes that distinguishing between treatment failure and re-infection is difficult. Tramont (1990) suggests a follow-up regimen of 3, 6 and 12 months for early and congenital syphilis to ensure that non-treponemal serology tests become negative or reach a very low titre and that there are no physical signs of infection. Also all patients with secondary syphilis should have a repeat test 2 years after treatment and anyone with documented neurosyphilis must be followed-up for 5 years.

Re-treatment may be indicated whenever clinical signs of syphilis continue or recur and whenever there is a sustained or an increased level in the VDRL titre or RPR. Careful follow-up is particularly important if the patient has had oral therapy (Thin, 1990).

Syphilis prevention and contact tracing

All patients with early acquired syphilis should be advised about contact tracing. First, the patient will need reassurance that the diagnosis and indeed the attendance at a GUM clinic will remain confidential. The patient must be informed that during the untreated primary and secondary stage of the disease, saliva, vaginal and seminal secretions are infectious (Tramont, 1990).

It is important to inform patients about their investigations and treatment and advise them to keep follow-up appointments, and also to explain fully to the patient that they are infectious and that their contacts should attend.

Primary and secondary syphilis are often referred to as early infectious syphilis. When early infectious syphilis is diagnosed, all sexual partners over the previous 6 months should be traced and examined as soon as possible, bearing in mind that full intercourse is not necessary for its transmission. Contact tracing is the preventive method that holds the greatest prospect of limiting the spread of venereal syphilis.

More patient education in terms of health promotion is necessary to eradicate syphilis altogether (Hook III, 1996). The use of barrier contraception and spermicidal preparations are effective measures against the transmission of syphilis, together with routine screening, case finding and adequate treatment of patients who are found to have the disease and their sexual partners.

Latent syphilis

Latent syphilis is the stage of the disease in which serological tests are positive, but in which there are no clinical manifestations of syphilis and the patient has not been treated (Robertson, McMillan & Young, 1989). CSF and chest X-ray films are normal. However, when this situation arises it does not imply a lack of progression of the disease, as further activity can occur at any time during latency. A full history should be sought from the patient, to find out if there are any details compatible with primary or secondary syphilis, or if there has been any known exposure to a syphilitic person or delivery of an infant with congenital syphilis. The latent period of syphilis follows the secondary stage of the disease and is divided into early latent and late latent syphilis, depending on the length of time the disease has been present.

Early latent syphilis describes the disease that has been present for up to 2 years. Relapses may occur, when the patient is infectious, and more people are likely to have relapses in the first year of contracting syphilis, with the incidence decreasing in the years thereafter (Sparling, 1990).

Late latent syphilis is the term used to describe untreated syphilis that was acquired more than 2 years ago. It may persist for many years or even for life (Robertson, McMillan & Young, 1989). The patient is considered not to be infectious during this time unless relapses occur. However, a pregnant woman with late latent syphilis can infect her foetus *in utero* and infection can also be transmitted via transfused contaminated blood.

About one third of patients remain asymptomatic for the rest of their lives and another third eventually become seronegative to standard tests for syphilis. In these cases of biological cure, it is assumed that *T. pallidum* has been eliminated (Csonka & Oates, 1990). The remaining third go on to develop tertiary syphilis.

Robertson, McMillan and Young (1989) suggest that latent syphilis is probably the one seen most in late stage syphilis, because of the antibiotics people are given to treat other infections. Following diagnosis, the heart and great blood vessels are examined radiologically to exclude calcification in the aorta, and the CSF is tested to exclude CNS involvement.

Treatment and follow-up of latent syphilis

Latent syphilis present for less than a year should be treated with the same regimens as primary and secondary syphilis. If latent infection has been present for more than a year, the recommended regimens are benzathine penicillin 2.4 mega units by intramuscular injection once a week for 3 weeks (Benenson, 1990); aqueous procaine penicillin 600 000 IU by intramuscular injection daily for 15 days; or tetracycline 500 mg orally four times a day for 30 days (Csonka & Oates, 1990).

An essential part of management in the GUM clinic is to interview the patient and ensure that all the sexual partners at risk are examined, investigated and, if necessary, treated.

Tertiary (late syphilis)

Late or tertiary syphilis is a slow, progressive, inflammatory disease resulting from untreated syphilis. It can affect any organ in the body and can produce clinical illness years after the initial infection, though it is now rarely seen in the Western world. It is not infectious and can be treated, but there is no cure for the damage it has already done to the body (Oates, 1969).

It is referred to as neurosyphilis when the organisms have invaded the CNS – 10% of patients; cardiovascular syphilis when it affects the structures of the cardiovascular system – 10%; and gummatous syphilis when the organisms invade the brain, bone, skin and internal organs –15% (Adler, 1990).

Neurosyphilis

Prior to penicillin treatment, neurosyphilis played a major part of the syphilis disease process and mental hospitals were crowded with syphilitic patients whose mental and physical health was failing (Robertson, McMillan & Young, 1989), but as a result of the introduction of successful antibiotic treatments, neurosyphilis is rarely seen today. The term refers to the late stage of the illness, rather than to the invasion of the CNS that occurs during the early stages of the disease in 20–30% of patients (Csonka & Oates, 1990) and which may or may not lead to acute meningeal neurosyphilis. There is a higher incidence of neurosyphilis in men than in women and it affects Caucasians more than black races (Csonka & Oates, 1990). Swartz (1990) notes that deaths from end-stage neurosyphilis in the UK reduced from 600 annually in 1941 to 24 in 1968.

For descriptive purposes, late neurosyphilis is usually divided into asymptomatic and symptomatic phases. The diagnosis of asymptomatic neurosyphilis is given to patients who have no clinical manifestations of neurological disease, but have CSF abnormalities. These include 5 x 10^6/l or more white blood cells; an elevated protein, over 40 mg/100 ml; and usually a positive FTA-ABS response (Csonka & Oates, 1990). A high white cell count is indicative of a meningeal reaction and serological tests are positive. Csonka and Oates (1990) reported that 'asymptomatic neurosyphilis occurs in about 20% of untreated patients, 20% of whom progress to symptomatic neurosyphilis in the absence of treatment.'

Robertson, McMillan and Young (1989) indicate that pupillary abnormalities may be present and late asymptomatic neurosyphilis may occasionally be accompanied by evidence of syphilitic involvement of other organs. Symptomatic forms of neurosyphilis include meningovascular syphilis, parenchymatous neurosyphilis, tabes dorsalis and other forms of spinal syphilis.

Meningovascular neurosyphilis

Meningovascular neurosyphilis refers to the development of endarteritis obliterans, inflammation inside small arteries, that leads to their collapse and obstruction. It affects the small blood vessels of the meninges, brain and spinal cord and leads to multiple small areas of infarction. There may be third, sixth and eighth cranial nerve involvement and the main symptom is a headache. Adler (1990) describes cranial nerve palsies and pupillary abnormalities as manifestations of this stage. The pupil abnormality is known as the 'Argyll Robertson pupil', a small irregular pupil that accommodates to near vision but does not react to light or painful stimuli. Other symptoms include hemiplegia, aphasia, epilepsy and mental deterioration.

Parenchymatous neurosyphilis

Parenchymatous neurosyphilis includes general paresis and tabes dorsalis and it refers to the destruction of nerve cells, principally in the cerebral cortex. The former represents an inflammatory process and the latter a degenerative one, but a mixture of the two pathological processes is always present. Vascular involvement may lead to a wide spectrum of conditions, ranging from hemiplegia to progressive neurological deficits that are the result of the gradual destruction of nerve tissue by small vessel endarteritis.

General paresis

General paresis, otherwise known as dementia paralytica or general paralysis of the insane (GPI), is very rare today. Researchers note that it develops 10 to 20 years after the original infection, almost exclusively in men (Csonka & Oates, 1990). Early in this part of the disease process symptoms include memory loss, malaise and personality changes, headaches, tremors and insomnia. Then, later on, patients may suffer from dementia, delusions of grandeur and convulsions.

Tabes dorsalis

Spinal cord damage (tabes dorsalis) principally involves dysfunction of the posterior column, dorsal roots and dorsal root ganglia that eventually results in the development of an ataxic wide-based gait and footslap (Csonka & Oates, 1990). Paraesthesiae; shooting or lightning pains of sudden onset, rapid radiation and sudden disappearance; bladder disturbances; faecal incontinence; impotence; loss of position and vibratory sense; absent ankle and knee jerks; loss of deep pain and temperature sensation; a positive Romberg's sign – the inability to stand with feet together and eyes closed without falling over; degenerative joint disease or Charcot's joints; and traumatic ulcers or sores on the lower extremities and feet are all prominent features in the classical picture.

Tabes dorsalis is usually seen in patients between the ages of 35 and 55 years and it affects men four to five times more often than women (Csonka & Oates, 1990).

Three other special forms of neurosyphilis need to be mentioned for completeness: syphilitic otitis or asymmetric deafness, tinnitus and optic atrophy. In the early stages they are curable, but if untreated they cause irreversible damage. Tramont (1990) discusses how the ear or the eye may be involved during any stage of syphilis and can cause diagnostic dilemmas. Robertson, McMillan and Young (1989) suggest that up to one third of patients may be blinded as a result of optic atrophy, even with penicillin treatment.

There are numerous currently known conditions from which neurosyphilis must be differentiated. A few examples are alcoholic neuropathy, multiple sclerosis, Alzheimer's disease and, in fact, any other disorder affecting the CNS. In relation to the CNS, the axiom that syphilis can mimic any disease is particularly relevant (Tramont, 1990).

Diagnosis of neurosyphilis

The diagnosis of neurosyphilis is difficult without neurological signs and is therefore based on serological tests, CSF examination and clinical judgment. Though serological tests are useful in confirming the diagnosis of syphilis, non-treponemal serological tests for syphilis are not sensitive enough and can be negative in late stages of the disease. Of the serology tests, the FTA-ABS test on CSF seems to be the most specific and sensitive. Csonka and Oates (1990) confirm that if the CSF TPHA or FTA-ABS tests are negative, neurosyphilis can be excluded.

When patients have latent syphilis, a lumbar puncture is carried out to exclude neurosyphilis and while some GUM clinics may have facilities to carry out this procedure, it is not uncommon for patients to be admitted to a day ward within the hospital for this investigation. CSF is examined in the laboratory for the number of white cells, total protein, IgG estimation and the serological tests VDRL, FTA-ABS and TPHA (Adler, 1990). De Silva, Walzman and Shahmanesh (1991) suggest that the TPHA titre should be taken into consideration before arranging a lumbar puncture for a patient and that it should be at least 1 in 2560, especially if the patient is asymptomatic.

Tramont (1990) recommends that any patient found to have a positive serum TPHA test, a positive CSF-VDRL and/or evidence of local CNS antibody production, with or without otherwise explained neurologic findings, warrants treatment or close follow-up for neurosyphilis.

Treatment and follow-up of neurosyphilis

'The introduction of penicillin in the treatment of neurosyphilis strikingly simplified and improved the therapy and outcome in this disease' (Swartz, 1990), though it has not been clearly defined what minimum dose of penicillin is needed for adequate treatment of neurosyphilis (Goldmeier & Hay, 1993).

Benzathine penicillin 2.4 million units intramuscularly weekly for three doses has been thought to be adequate treatment for all forms of neurosyphilis (Swartz, 1990). However, Goldmeier and Hay (1993) do not agree and instead recommend procaine penicillin 1.8 or 2.4 million units intramuscularly daily with probenecid 0.5 g orally 6- hourly for 21 days. They also note that in penicillin allergy, doxycycline 200–400 mg per day for 28 days may be prescribed.

Csonka and Oates (1990) recommend that clinical and CSF examination should be performed 4 weeks after antibiotic treatment of patients with neurosyphilis. The examination should be repeated after 2 months and 12 months if the patient is improving clinically and the cell count is falling. Serological tests on serum should be performed at 6 and 12 months and then at yearly intervals for 3 years. Untreated, general paresis is progressive and fatal. The prognosis of tabes dorsalis is variable and the disease process can halt at an early stage.

Cardiovascular syphilis

Syphilis was a major cause of cardiovascular disease 100 years ago, but today it is relatively uncommon. Nevertheless, syphilitic heart disease may present without warning in late latent syphilis and needs to be considered in patients with aortic or aortic valve disease (Healy, 1990). *T. pallidum* is believed to spread to the heart during the early stages of infection, possibly via the lymphatics and the lymph nodes. The organisms lodge in the aortic wall where they remain dormant for years.

Cardiovascular disease processes start early in the course of untreated syphilis and it appears to affect more men than women (Csonka & Oates, 1990), with clinical presentation appearing between 40 and 55 years of age (Healy, 1990). The aorta is most commonly affected by aortitis, which may be uncomplicated and asymptomatic or may cause an aneurysm of the aorta or ascending aortic regurgitation. Smaller vessels may also be affected and aneurysms of carotid and subclavian vessels have also been noted (Adler, 1990).

During the early stages of cardiovascular syphilis, the patient is asymptomatic but as the disease progresses, the signs and symptoms are no different from other causes of cardiac disease and the patient may present with angina, left ventricular failure or paroxysmal nocturnal dyspnoea (Adler, 1990).

Diagnosis and treatment of cardiovascular syphilis

Csonka and Oates (1990) suggest that diagnostic procedures in the assessment of a patient with cardiovascular disease include a chest X-ray to show the arch of the aorta and screening to detect aortic dilatation. An electrocardiogram and cardiac catheterisation may also be indicated.

Antibiotic therapy should be administered as early as possible. Csonka and Oates (1990) recommend a course of procaine penicillin 600 000 IU intramuscularly daily for 20 days, or tetracycline or erythromycin 500 mg orally four times a day for 30 days. Congestive cardiac failure should be treated before penicillin is given, but the prognosis is not good (Csonka & Oates, 1990).

A cardiac surgeon should be consulted before treatment commences, as surgery in the form of aortic valve replacement or coronary artery bypass grafting may be indicated. The prognosis of patients with cardiovascular syphilis depends on the extent of the disease and the patient's general wellbeing (Csonka & Oates, 1990). Robertson, McMillan and Young (1989) suggest that the mortality rate in surgery for aneurysms of the ascending aorta may be as high as 40%.

Chest pain and sudden death often occur in patients with cardio-vascular syphilitic disease (Healy, 1990). Unfortunately, because it is not an active infection and degenerative changes have already taken place around the heart, antibiotic therapy does not serve much purpose.

Gummatous syphilis

Late benign syphilis represents an inflammatory process that can occur anywhere in the body but most commonly in the skeletal system, skin and mucocutaneous tissues. Incidence of gummatous syphilis decreased steadily over many years as a result of the treatment of early and latent syphilis, even before penicillin therapy was introduced (Kampmeier, 1990).

The gumma is a granulomatous lesion occurring in late syphilis, 3 to 12 years after the primary infection (Adler, 1990). It closely resembles the lesion of tuberculosis; the term 'gumma' refers to the necrotic debris in the lesion which is of a gummy consistency (Kampmeier, 1990). Gummas may occur singly or in groups and vary in size (Tramont, 1990). On the skin, gummas start as painless nodules, which break down into one or more punched out ulcers. Due to slough, the base may have a 'wash leather' appearance (Robertson, McMillan & Young, 1989). It heals slowly from the centre, taking weeks or months and the resulting scar is like thin tissue paper. This combination of atrophy and pigmentary changes can be of considerable retrospective diagnostic value.

Gummata occur mostly on the lower leg, face and scalp. Gummas of the bone are about as common as gummas of the skin and may result in fractures or joint destruction (Kampmeier, 1990). Osteoporosis of long bones, especially of the tibia and fibula, causes thickening of the bones and unlike most other syphilitic lesions is often painful.

Mucocutaneous gummata infrequently affect the mouth and throat. Lesions of the palate may lead to local destruction and eventual perforation. When the hard palate and the nasal septum are affected, there is generally involvement of the underlying bone. Gummata of the pharynx and larynx produce symptoms such as hoarseness or dysphagia, and stenosis or severe deformity may result (Kampmeier, 1990).

Where a testis is affected, gummatous infiltration and dense fibrosis produce a smooth, painless enlargement, which is also painless on palpation. The testis has to be surgically removed to exclude testicular cancer (Robertson, McMillann & Young, 1989). The liver is the most commonly affected internal organ, though this is extremely rare today, and lesions of other internal organs have also been reported (Adler, 1990).

Diagnosis and treatment of gummatous syphilis

Serological tests are usually reactive, especially when there is involvement of soft tissue (Kampmeier, 1990). Treponemes are difficult to visualise on microscopy (Tramont, 1990), though mouth lesions should be biopsied as malignant changes are common (Robertson, McMillan & Young, 1989).

Csonka and Oates (1990) recommend procaine penicillin 600 000 IU intramuscularly daily for 15 days. They note that when treating patients with gumma of the larynx, some physicians prescribe oral corticosteroids to cover the first injection of penicillin, in an attempt to minimise any JHR reaction.

Syphilis during pregnancy

Although uncommon, syphilis remains a serious disease, especially during pregnancy when it may result in significant perinatal morbidity and mortality. Untreated primary or secondary syphilis in pregnant women can lead to symptomatic congenital syphilis or intrauterine death, though some babies escape infection (Csonka & Oates, 1990). Congenital syphilis is a preventable disease if maternal infection is diagnosed early and treated with penicillin.

Transmission of treponemes to the foetus occurs more often when the mother's infection is in the early stage, the probability being 80–90% during the first year of maternal infection (Robertson, McMillan & Young, 1989). After that the chances decline and after the fourth year it is rare.

Diagnosis and treatment

Diagnosis in the pregnant patient is made in the same way as in the non-pregnant patient. Screening for syphilis after the first 3 months of pregnancy is a well established practice in Europe, the USA and Australia (Boot et al., 1992). However, infection can occur after screening has taken place, and this can result in congenital syphilis. In areas where syphilis is still endemic, Qolohle et al. (1995) recommend rescreening at the time of delivery. Following a diagnosis of latent syphilis in a pregnant woman, it is important to try and confirm the duration of infection and rule out prior treatment. The pregnant patient should also be carefully examined for other STDs.

Treatment should be initiated as early as possible. As a JHR reaction is more likely to happen after the first penicillin injection for early syphilis, it is possible for a JHR in the second or third trimester to induce uterine contractions resulting in premature labour (Zenker & Rolfs, 1990). Therefore, if a woman notices a reduction in foetal movements during treatment or if other symptoms occur, she should be seen by an obstetrician immediately.

Tramont (1990) notes that the treatment of syphilis in pregnancy is related to the stage of the disease and follows the treatment schedule described before.

Pregnant women with syphilis who are allergic to penicillin present a therapeutic challenge. Erythromycin, which has a high cure rate in the adult with early syphilis, may not prevent congenital syphilis (Tramont, 1990). Tetracycline, which is also effective in the non-pregnant patient, is generally not recommended for pregnant women because of possible yellow-brown discoloration of foetal deciduous teeth if the drug is given in the second half of pregnancy (Boot et al., 1992). Robertson, McMillan and Young (1989) suggest that penicillin desensitisation may be considered and if not readily available, ceftriaxone 1 g may be given intramuscularly for 14 days, although there is not much data available on the effectiveness of ceftriaxone in treating the foetus or its use during pregnancy to prevent congenital syphilis (Tramont, 1990).

Once the diagnosis of syphilis is confirmed and active treatment started, immediate contact tracing of the patient's partner(s) is very important. This protects the patient from possible re-infection and limits further spread of the disease. The seriousness of the situation should be explained to the patient and it should also be stressed that the disease is curable and that there should not be any harmful effects on the baby. It is essential to remember though, that even in situations where full and adequate treatment has been administered to the patient, foetal involvement may occur, resulting in congenital syphilis.

Congenital syphilis

It is well established that *T. pallidum* can readily cross the placental barrier, especially when a syphilitic mother is in the early stage of the disease (Robertson, McMillan & Young, 1989). The later in pregnancy the mother acquires the infection, the more severe the infection will be in the foetus. Congenital syphilis can have devastating consequences, for example mental deficiency, chronic meningitis, blindness and deafness, though it rarely occurs in Britain nowadays as pregnant women have a reactive blood test during their antenatal care.

The incidence of congenital syphilis decreased throughout the Western world in the 1970s and early 1980s, but there was a rise again in the mid-1980s in Australia and the USA, along with a higher incidence of syphilis in the heterosexual population (Csonka & Oates, 1990). In the UK, just over 50 cases of congenital syphilis were reported from GUM clinics in 1994 (DOH, 1995).

When it occurs, congenital syphilis is classified into early, latent and late stages. In the early stage, the condition is infectious and resembles acquired secondary syphilis in many ways. Infants usually appear perfectly healthy at birth, then fail to thrive and clinical signs start to appear 2–12 weeks after birth (Robertson, McMillan & Young, 1989). Clinical features may include a widespread rash extending to the palms of the hands and soles of the feet. The secondary rash may be seen between the buttocks, and may be crusted or red and ulcerated.

Robertson, McMillan and Young (1989) also suggest that condylomata lata may appear in moist skin areas; the skin becomes yellowish and the child appears wasted with an ageing appearance and there may be patchy hair loss.

Mucous patches appear in the nose, mouth, throat and larynx, which gives rise to rhinitis, and lymphatic glands may be enlarged with distension of the abdomen and spleen (Csonka & Oates, 1990). Bones may be affected, giving rise to painful joints and apparent paralysis of the joints, and if there is involvement of the CNS, convulsions may occur (Robertson, McMillan & Young, 1989) and there may be retarded development of the brain resulting in mental abnormality.

At birth, a necrotising funicitis or damage to the umbilical cord may be seen, which is diagnostic of congenital syphilis (Tramont, 1990). Dark-field microscopy from skin lesions or nasal discharge can establish the diagnosis immediately and positive serological tests for syphilis are confirmatory.

If syphilitic children survive the first year of life, they enter a latent period (Tramont, 1990) and are not infectious. Lesions that appear for the first time after the child's second birthday constitute late congenital syphilis (Csonka & Oates, 1990). The manifestations of late syphilis include gummata, involving the skin, bone, mucous membrane and viscera as described for acquired syphilis. Nasal deformities occur as a result of destruction of the nasal septum (Tramont, 1990).

Interstitial keratitis may occur as late as 30 years of age and it may affect one or both eyes, appearing suddenly with pain, photophobia and blurred vision, the attack may resolve itself or recur and each attack leaves a corneal scar resulting in impaired vision (Robertson, McMillan & Young, 1989).

There may be a gradual loss of hearing and in some cases complete deafness when the eighth cranial nerve is affected. Neurosyphilis is a more common phenomenon in congenital syphilis than in acquired syphilis, affecting 15% or more of children with late symptomatic disease (Csonka & Oates, 1990). A degree of tabes dorsalis may occur.

Sometimes other gross stigmata of the disease are present and these defects are caused by deformities from healed lesions. They include destruction of the nasal bones, giving rise to a flattened bridge or 'saddle nose', a high and arched palate, and a prominent maxillary bone and notching of the cerebral incisors with thickening of the teeth from front to back (Robertson, McMillan & Young, 1989), giving them a barrel-shaped appearance.

The treatment in early congenital syphilis is benzyl or procaine penicillin 50 000 units/kg body weight for 10 days and in late congenital syphilis, the treatment is as for the equivalent stage in late latent acquired syphilis (Robertson, McMillan & Young, 1989).

Monitoring of treatment of syphilis in both mother and baby is required for a period of at least 2 years. The importance of follow-up after treatment cannot be over-emphasised. The RPR or VDRL tests should show titres falling progressively and not rising again and Robertson, McMillan and Young (1989) believe that retreatment should be given if there is a four-fold rise in titre levels.

References

Adler MW (1990) ABC of Sexually Transmitted Diseases, 2nd edn. London: British Medical Association.

Aral SO (1996) The social context of syphilis persistence in the south-eastern United States. Sexually Transmitted Diseases 23(1): 9–15.

Benenson AS (1990) Control of Communicable Diseases in Man, 15th edn. Washington: American Public Health Association.

Boot JM, Oranje AP, De Groot R, Tan G, Stolz E (1992) Congenital syphilis. International Journal of STD & AIDS 3: 161–7.

Caffyn-Parsons U (1978) Venereal diseases. Nursing Mirror Supplement (May 25): i–iv.

Chang SN, Chung K-Y, Lee M-G, Lee JB (1995) Seroconversion of the serological tests for syphilis in the newborns born to treated syphilitic mothers. Genitourinary Medicine 71: 68–70.

Csonka GW, Oates JK (1990) Syphilis. In Csonka GW, Oates JK (Eds), Sexually Transmitted Diseases – A Textbook of Genitourinary Medicine. London: Baillière Tindall.

De Silva, Walzman M, Shahmanesh (1991) The value of serum TPHA titres in selecting patients for lumbar puncture. Genitourinary Medicine 67: 37–40.

DOH (1995) Sexually Transmitted Diseases, England 1994. Department of Health Statistical Bulletin. London: HMSO.

El-Zaatari MM, Martens MG (1994) False-negative screening due to change in temperature. Sexually Transmitted Diseases 21(5): 243–5.

Evans G (1994) A history of sexually transmitted diseases. Nursing Times 90(18): 29–31.

Goeman J, Kivuv UM, Nzila N, Behets F, Edidi B, Gnaore E, Van Dyck E, St Louis M, Piot P, Laga M (1995) Similar serological response to conventional therapy for syphilis among HIV-positive and HIV-negative women. Genitourinary Medicine 71: 275–9.

Goldmeier D, Hay P (1993) A review and update on adult syphilis, with particular reference to its treatment. International Journal of STD & AIDS 4: 70–82.

Healy BP (1990) Cardiovascular syphilis. In Holmes KK, Mårdh P-A, Sparling PF, Wiesner PJ (Eds), Sexually Transmitted Diseases, 2nd edn. New York: McGraw-Hill.

Hook III EW (1996) Biomedical issues in syphilis control. Sexually Transmitted Diseases 23(1): 5–8.

Kampmeier RH (1990) Late benign syphilis. In Holmes KK, Mårdh P-A, Sparling PF, Wiesner PJ (Eds), Sexually Transmitted Diseases, 2nd edn. New York: McGraw-Hill.

Linglöf T (1995) Rapid increase of syphilis and gonorrhoea in parts of the former USSR. Sexually Transmitted Diseases 22(3): 160–1.

Musher DM (1990) Biology of *Treponema pallidum*. In Holmes KK, Mårdh P-A, Sparling PF, Wiesner PJ (Eds), Sexually Transmitted Diseases, 2nd edn. New York: McGraw-Hill.

Oates JK (1969) The sexually transmitted diseases. Nursing Mirror February 7: 24–7.

Qolohle DC, Hoosen AA, Moodley J, Smith AN, Mlisana KP (1995) Serological screening for sexually transmitted infections in pregnancy: is there any value in re-screening for HIV and syphilis at the time of delivery? Genitourinary Medicine 71: 65–7.

Robertson DHH, McMillan A, Young H (1989) Clinical Practice in Sexually Transmissible Diseases, 2nd edn. Edinburgh: Churchill Livingstone.

Savall R, Valls F, Cabre M (1991) Syphilis and HIV infection. Genitourinary Medicine 67: 353.

Schmid G (1996) Serologic screening for syphilis: rationale, cost and realpolitik. Sexually Transmitted Diseases 23(1): 45–50.

Smikle MF, James OB'L, Prabhakar P (1990) Biological false positive serological tests for syphilis in the Jamaican population. Genitourinary Medicine 66: 76–8.

Sparling PF (1990) Natural history of syphilis. In Holmes KK, Mårdh P-A, Sparling PF, Wiesner PJ (Eds), Sexually Transmitted Diseases, 2nd edn. New York: McGraw-Hill.

St Louis ME, Farley TA, Aral SO (1996) Untangling the persistence of syphilis in the south. Sexually Transmitted Diseases 23(1): 1–4.

Swartz MN (1990) Neurosyphilis. In Holmes KK, Mårdh P-A, Sparling PF, Wiesner PJ (Eds), Sexually Transmitted Diseases, 2nd edn. New York: McGraw-Hill.

Thin RN (1990) Early syphilis in the adult. In Holmes KK, Mårdh P-A, Sparling PF, Wiesner PJ (Eds), Sexually Transmitted Diseases, 2nd edn. New York: McGraw-Hill.

Tramont EC (1990) *Treponema pallidum* (syphilis). In Mandell GL, Douglas RG, Bennett JE (Eds), Principles and Practice of Infectious Diseases. New York: Churchill Livingstone.

Waugh M (1991) The great pox. International Journal of STD & AIDS 2 (supplement 1): 26–9.

Zenker PN, Rolfs RT (1990) Treatment of syphilis, 1989. Reviews of Infectious Diseases 12 (supplement 6): S590–S609.

THE LIBRARY
KENT & SUSSEX HOSPITAL
TUNBRIDGE WELLS
KENT TN4 8AT

Chapter 5
Gonorrhoea and non-specific urethritis

Pauline Handy

Gonorrhoea

History

Gonorrhoea is an infection that has been known for thousands of years; descriptions of it have been found in the Old Testament of the Bible. References to the infection can also be found in Chinese, Egyptian and Greek literature. Indeed, the word gonorrhoea comes from the Greek word meaning 'flow of seed'. Writing in 130 AD, Galen postulated that the urethral discharge present with the infection was in fact semen – hence seed (Hook III & Handsfield, 1990). Little attention appears to have been given to women infected with gonorrhoea, presumably because many of them were asymptomatic. However the part played by women in the transmission of gonorrhoea was understood and Moses gave clear instructions on how to control its spread (Oates & Csonka, 1990). In Leviticus Chapter 15 in the Bible, Moses was given detailed instructions by God about hygiene and cleanliness in men with a discharge or 'issue', to prevent contamination of both objects such as bedding and clothes and of their women.

More recently, gonorrhoea has been known as the clap; the first reference to the clap dates back to 1378. It is thought that the word clap came from the name of a district in Paris, where prostitutes gathered in the Middle Ages. The area became known as Les Clapier.

Sherrard and Bingham (1995) suggest that worldwide there are now around 200 million cases of gonorrhoea a year.

The gonococcus

The bacterial infective agent for gonorrhoea is a member of the genus *Neisseriae*, named after Neisser, who discovered it in 1879. Its appearance on Gram staining is of Gram-negative or red-stained kidney bean shaped diplococci, which always appear in pairs with the concavities facing each other. These are usually found within pus cells (polymorphs) and are therefore often referred to as intracellular Gram-negative diplococci.

Gonorrhoea commonly affects the urethra, cervix, rectum and oropharynx. Rare sites of infection include blood, skin, joints and conjunctiva.

Neisseria meningitidis is another member of the *Neisseria* genus which may be found in the nasopharynx, rectum or cervix, though the patient is often asymptomatic and isolation of this organism is usually of no significance. It is only possible to determine which strain of gonorrhoea is present by culturing specimens in the laboratory.

Gonorrhoea, together with syphilis and chancre, is a venereal disease with a statutory requirement for reporting to the Centre for Disease Surveillance and Control (CDSC), which correlates reports from around the country and produces infection statistics for monitoring the spread of infection.

Transmission and prevalence

To date, gonorrhoea has only been found in humans and the most usual mode of transmission has been found to be through sexual intercourse or close physical contact. Sparling (1990) notes that gonococci are only viable outside the human body for a short time and that there is almost no evidence that gonorrhoea can be passed on from toilet seats or such like. In order to facilitate transmission, close physical contact with infected mucosa is required and the risk of infection from a single episode with an infected partner has been calculated at 60–90% for females and 20–50% for males (Sherrard & Bingham, 1995).

It is possible, although not common, for an infected person to transfer gonorrhoea from their genital area to their eyes or their partner's eyes via fingers or possibly towels, which may lead to a gonococcal conjunctivitis (Oates & Csonka, 1990). An infected mother may also infect the eyes of her baby as the child passes through the birth canal at delivery, giving rise to a condition known as ophthalmia neonatorum. However, such cases are fairly uncommon in the UK and the most usual mode of transmission remains sexual intercourse.

The disease is highly infectious, with women more at risk of being infected by their male partners than the other way round (Oates & Csonka, 1990), because the female anatomy has a much greater area of mucosa available. This makes prevention difficult unless condoms are used, especially as gonococci are known to penetrate mucosal surfaces and colonise the submucosal layer.

The number of gonorrhoea infections in Britain has fallen steadily since 1977 and there was a particularly big decrease in 1987 (Bignell, 1994). However, in poorer nations, the infection is still fairly widespread, probably through lack of facilities for treatment and contact tracing, as well as lack of effective health education (Sherrard & Bingham, 1995).

In the UK, *The Health of the Nation* document (DOH, 1993) set a target of reducing gonorrhoea from 61 to less than 49 new cases per 100 000 of the population aged 15–64 by 1995, and most Genito-Urinary Medicine (GUM) clinics appear to have achieved this target.

Incubation period

The average incubation period for gonorrhoea is 3–7 days after exposure to the infection, although it must be remembered that symptoms may present at any time between 1 and 14 days after exposure. However, many women and some men are asymptomatic, which makes it difficult to estimate an incubation period for all cases.

It is essential that when taking swabs from patients the nurse bears in mind the incubation period of gonorrhoea. Many GUM clinics take a second set of tests, generally a minimum of a week after the first set, to check for infection that may not have been seen the first time. Other clinics only take a second set of tests if symptoms are present at the time of the return visit.

Incubation periods are important when the patient is seen by the health adviser or nurse as he or she will be able to work out which partners, if any, have been put at most risk of infection. Asymptomatic infection poses a greater problem to the health adviser or nurse for contact tracing, as the patient may not be aware of when the infection was acquired.

Testing for gonorrhoea

Mårdh and Danielsson (1990) suggest that although the use of microscopy has great benefit in diagnosing gonorrhoea and showing up the presence or absence of inflammation, cultures should always be taken because of the problems of microscopic diagnosis with asymptomatic patients.

Gonococci may be less obvious on microscopy in female patients than in males, because in the female, gonococci often present in single pairs rather than groups, making them much more difficult to identify, especially if the patient has a concurrent infection such as bacterial vaginosis. Andrews et al. (1994) investigated doing microscopy on samples from women only if they complained of symptoms such as discharge, soreness, itching, etc., or if the clinician noted a discharge or the women were contacts of patients with gonorrhoea. They concluded that selective microscopy was effective and safe and could be more efficient, as it allowed laboratory staff more time for specimens from patients with a probable problem.

It has been estimated that the sensitivity of microscopy in detecting gonorrhoea from the cervix is only 50–65% (Oates & Csonka, 1990), though a slightly higher figure of 66.7% in 1993 was noted by Edwards and Dockerty (1995). One would expect to find a large number of polymorphs on the cervical or urethral slides, indicating that an infection was present. This is due to the gonococci initiating an intense inflammatory response, resulting in the production of large numbers of polymorphs.

High vaginal secretions fail to show gonococci as the infection has not been found to colonise this area. Instead gonococci are attracted to areas of columnar epithelium, which are found on the cervix, urethra, rectum and conjuctiva. Therefore, when taking swabs from a female patient for examination under the microscope, the urethra and cervix are the areas of choice to sample. Mårdh and Danielsson (1990) note that some ingredients, in what they describe as gynaecological exploration cream, have been shown to kill gonococci and therefore the speculum used should just be warmed with warm water.

In male patients, swabs should be taken from the urethra for microscopical examination and again large amounts of polymorphs will be evident, together with clusters of Gram-negative intracellular diplococci. It has been suggested that up to 98% of infection in the male urethra can be isolated on microscopy (Sherrard & Bingham, 1995), though Edwards and Dockerty (1995) noted a microscopic diagnosis rate in men of 91.7% in 1993.

Evans et al. (1994) suggest that rectal specimens from either sex of patient should be taken from mucosa clear of faeces, to avoid contaminating the specimen with faecal organisms.

Diagnosis should always be confirmed by samples cultured in the laboratory. Various culture media are now available for this purpose and one that is frequently used is New York culture medium, while another common one is Thayer-Martin. Carbon dioxide is needed to encourage growth of the organism on culture medium and specimens should be placed in a carbon dioxide incubator with a concentration of 3–10% carbon dioxide. If laboratory facilities are not available, the use of a transport medium such as Stuart's transport medium is acceptable, as this allows the growth of gonococci up to 48 hours after collection (Oates & Csonka, 1990). Figure 5.1 shows how gonococci and polymorphs appear on microscopy slides.

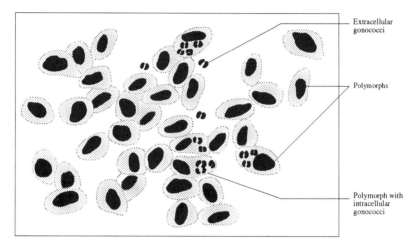

Extracellular gonococci

Polymorphs

Polymorph with intracellular gonococci

Figure 5.1: Gonococci and polymorphs on a microscopy slide

The two-glass urine test is a non-invasive, extremely simple and inexpensive test carried out in most GUM clinics to help identify infection, and all men attending GUM departments should be asked to do a two-glass urine test. The urine may be examined visually as described in Chapter 1, Figure 1.9; and also under the microscope if threads or specks are present. The nurse may be able to see multiple polymorphs on microscopy, which would indicate infection. The two-glass urine test cannot be used to differentiate between gonococcal and non-gonococcal urethritis. Laboratory dipsticks of the urine may show a raised level of white cells indicating the need for further investigations.

Ross (1996) observed that the use of serotyping of gonococcal isolates to find different serovars may help a clinician find out whether a re-infection is from a new partner or the same partner, though if the same serotype is predominant in a particular geographical area this method may be of no use. He also notes that serotyping may be of use in cases of rape or sexual abuse. Ross et al. (1994) found that different serovars were associated with particular patterns of sexual behaviour, that is heterosexually or homosexually acquired gonorrhoea, and they also noted differences in the serovars found in different cities.

Auxotyping is another method of classifying strains of gonor-rhoea and is useful in epidemiological studies (Mårdh & Danielsson, 1990).

Clinical features in female patients

It is important to remember that many women infected with gonor-rhoea will remain asymptomatic and the practitioner should not be misled by the lack of symptoms. Barlow and Phillips (1978) found 40% of female patients with gonorrhoea to be asymptomatic.

Women often have a vaginal discharge which they consider to be normal and not worthy of mentioning when the history is being taken. The discharge may be caused by conditions such as thrush or bacterial vaginosis and the possibility of infection with gonorrhoea may be overlooked unless the patient is forthcoming about her sexual history. If a large number of polymorphs are seen on the cervical specimen during microscopy, it is prudent to take swabs from the patient for both gonorrhoea and chlamydia, if these have not already been obtained.

The patient may complain of dysuria and frequency caused by urethritis, due to infection with gonorrhoea, and she may have a purulent discharge from her urethra. A urethral swab should be taken, though the urethra may sometimes need to be milked to encourage the expulsion of exudate for examination (Mårdh & Danielsson, 1990). This is done by using one finger in the vagina to gently stroke upwards and outwards under the urethra.

The cervix may look unremarkable or a cervicitis may be noted. Yellow or green discharge may be observed coming from the os. However, when urethritis and cervicitis are seen together, this is suggestive of gonorrhoea (Oates & Csonka, 1990). Patients may also complain of abdominal pain and backache and occasionally inflam-mation of the Bartholin's glands may be seen. The patient may also present with intermenstrual bleeding.

In general, the most common site for infection with gonorrhoea in women is the cervix, with around 90% of patients found to have cervical gonorrhoea (Barlow & Phillips, 1978). Gonorrhoea may also be found in the throats, rectums or urethras of women. Urethral infection can be found in about 73% of women with gonorrhoea (Thin & Shaw, 1979). Women may present with a gonococcal infection of more than one area and if there is any doubt about the risk of pharyngeal or rectal involvement, swabs should be taken to exclude the presence of gonorrhoea. The nurse should be sensitive to the feelings of the patient in all aspects of screening for sexually transmitted diseases (STDs). Asking a patient if she has had oral or anal intercourse is a difficult task, bearing in mind the possible distress of the patient and the unfortunate stigma that still surrounds STDs.

Rectal gonorrhoea has been found in nearly 40% of women and pharyngeal gonorrhoea in nearly 6% (Barlow & Phillips, 1978). Oral intercourse would now seem to be accepted as normal sexual behaviour, while anal intercourse may not be. The patient may become distressed when asked about anal intercourse and the nurse should take care to explain that rectal infection with gonorrhoea may occur even when anal intercourse has not taken place, as the female anatomy allows secretions to be transferred from the vagina to the rectum quite easily. Kinghorn and Rashid (1979) suggest that where there is rectal gonorrhoea in women, autoinoculation from infected vaginal discharge is very common.

Clinical features in male patients

The most common sign of gonorrhoea infection in men is acute anterior urethritis, and the majority of patients will complain of discharge and dysuria, although a small proportion will be asymptomatic (Hook III & Handsfield, 1990). If a patient does complain of discharge it will usually be profuse, purulent and either yellow or green in colour.

The dysuria is often described by those infected with gonorrhoea as like 'trying to pass broken glass' and it is extremely uncomfortable. For many patients, this is the first symptom that they notice. The meatus may become inflamed and swollen and occasionally the inguinal lymph nodes are inflamed.

Men with rectal gonorrhoea rarely report any symptoms, although they may complain of a vague perianal itch, soreness or discharge. On examination using a proctoscope, the rectal walls may be seen to be reddened and inflamed, though Oates and Csonka (1990) also state that the rectum may appear normal in some cases.

Oropharyngeal gonorrhoea may cause the patient to complain of a sore throat, but the infection is usually asymptomatic. Hook III and Handsfield (1990) suggest that the role played by pharyngeal gonorrhoea is uncertain.

In men, gonorrhoea has been found to colonise the urethra, oropharynx and anorectum, though rectal gonorrhoea is normally only found in homosexuals and in 40% of homosexual men, gonorrhoea is only isolated from the rectum (Sherrard & Bingham, 1995). It is always prudent to take specimens from the rectum, throat and urethra of homosexual men in view of their sexual behaviour. Pharyngeal infection is found in 10–25% of homosexual men and 3–7% of heterosexual men (Hook III & Handsfield, 1990). Oates and Csonka (1990) state that oropharyngeal infection in men is only found when oral sex has taken place.

Gonorrhoea in infants and children

Infants born to mothers infected with gonorrhoea may be born with sticky eyes, a condition known as ophthalmia neonatorum, which is legally defined as a purulent discharge from the eyes within the first 21 days after birth (Oates & Csonka, 1990). They also note that if left untreated, small areas of the conjunctiva may be destroyed, leading to possible ulceration of the cornea. In less developed areas of the world, blindness following infection with gonorrhoea is still a regular occurrence. Gutman and Wilfert (1990) suggest that nowadays in the developed world, gonorrhoea is one of the least common causes of ophthalmia neonatorum and chlamydia one of the most common.

The infection normally becomes obvious within a few days of delivery and examination of the discharge from the eye by microscopy after Gram staining or on culture will reveal the presence of gonococci. Gutman and Wilfert (1990) also note that oropharyngeal infection is found in about 35% of babies with gonococcal ophthalmia.

In 1881, Credé started using 2% silver nitrate drops as a prophylactic treatment and the rate of ophthalmia neonatorum dropped from 10 to 0.3% (Gutman & Wilfert, 1990), though Laga et al. (1988) have shown that 1% tetracycline ointment is just as effective for prophylaxis. Nowadays, prophylaxis has been stopped in most European countries, due to the low incidence of gonococcal ophthalmia (Oates & Csonka, 1990) and treatment, where infection is found, is with penicillin.

If a pregnant woman is found to have gonorrhoea, it is obviously important that she is treated to prevent infection in her baby and also reduce the risk of a premature birth or a low birthweight baby, both of which have been shown to be connected with gonorrhoea during pregnancy (Donders et al., 1993).

Gonorrhoea in children occurs more often in girls than boys and though urethral infection in boys is due to sexual activity, in girls infection in the vulvovaginal area may be from non-sexual contact with a parent or shared flannels or towels (Oates & Csonka, 1990). Gutman and Wilfert (1990) stress that sexual abuse should always be considered in prepubertal children with gonorrhoea. Vulvovaginal disease may lead to staining of underwear and inflammation and discharge may be found on examination, though specimens should be taken without the use of a speculum (Oates & Csonka, 1990). Treatment is with penicillin or a different regimen if penicillin-resistant gonorrhoea is prevalent in the area (Gutman & Wilfert, 1990).

Complications in females

Sherrard and Bingham (1995) note that there is a low rate of complications in men and women with gonorrhoea in the UK, which is probably partly due to the fact that diagnosis and treatment is fairly easy to access, but also the nature of the organism seems to have changed.

Bartholinitis and abscess

Hook III and Handsfield (1990) note that Bartholin's abscess is a common complication in women with gonorrhoea and suggest that routine urethral and cervical swabs for gonorrhoea should always be taken when a patient presents with Bartholinitis. The pressure on the Bartholin's ducts may result in pus being expelled and the diagnosis may be made. An abscess may develop and this often causes swelling of the vulval area and severe pain (Oates & Csonka, 1990). The diagnosis is normally based on Gramstain findings on microscopy and clinical examination, which can show a tender inflamed mass.

If this condition is caught in the early stages, a course of antibiotics can be successful as treatment. However, Oates and Csonka (1990) suggest that urgent surgery is usually needed to drain the abscess and marsupialise the gland, which involves the gland being stitched in such a way that an abscess cannot reform. Antibiotics also need to be given, often penicillin for at least 4 days.

Pelvic inflammatory disease

Pelvic inflammatory disease (PID) is potentially the most serious complication of infection with gonorrhoea. Oates and Csonka

(1990) suggest that an estimated 10% of women with gonorrhoea go on to develop PID, though Sherrard and Bingham (1995) suggest a much lower rate of around 1%. More detailed information about PID can be found in Chapter 6.

Complications in males

Epididymitis

The epididymis lies at the upper part of the testis and acts as a storehouse for sperm. Epididymitis or inflammation of the epididymis is the most common complication associated with gonorrhoea in men, though Oates and Csonka (1990) suggest that nowadays only 1% of men with gonorrhoea develop it. The patient may present with one-sided pain and swelling of the scrotal sac and show signs of urethritis, such as urethral discharge and dysuria (Hook III & Handsfield, 1990). On examination, a tender swelling of the epididymis will be present (Csonka & Oates, 1990). A scrotal support often brings relief to the patient and should be provided routinely (Adler, 1990); treatment with doxycycline has been suggested as effective.

Cowperitis and Tysonitis

Inflammation of the Cowper's glands is rarely seen these days in developed countries but can be more common in the Third World (Oates & Csonka, 1990). The patient may complain of frequency, perineal pain and severe pain on defecation, and on rectal examination the glands will feel hard and be extremely painful, as an abscess often forms in this area (Oates & Csonka, 1990).

The glands of Tyson are situated on either side of the frenum and may become inflamed, causing the glands to be swollen and hard to the touch, though treatment for gonorrhoea will normally clear up this condition (Oates & Csonka, 1990).

Prostatitis

Prostatitis is rarely seen these days because modern treatments are so effective. Adler (1990) notes that prostatitis relating to infection with gonorrhoea is normally an acute condition causing frequency, urgency, dysuria and fever rather than pain. Chronic prostatitis following gonorrhoea is commonly due to non-specific infection (Oates & Csonka, 1990) or chlamydia, and the main problem it causes is pain, which may occur in many places in the genital area and sometimes after ejaculation (Adler, 1990). He also suggests that treatment should be with an antibiotic such as doxycycline or erythromycin as these penetrate into prostatic tissue.

Urethral stricture and periurethral abscess

Both of these conditions are now very rare in the UK as antibiotic treatment is so good (Hook III & Handsfield, 1990), though Oates and Csonka (1990) note that strictures are seen in tropical countries. Strictures are probably caused by repeated infections or the urethral irrigation that used to be done as treatment for gonorrhoea before antibiotics were available (Hook III & Handsfield, 1990).

Disseminated infection

The most common systemic complication of gonorrhoea is usually a disseminated infection, with the patient presenting with acute arthritis and/or dermatitis (Hook III & Handsfield, 1990). Adler (1990) suggests that disseminated gonococcal infection (DGI) is a rare complication and Oates and Csonka (1990) feel it only affects about 1% of patients nowadays, with more women than men affected, probably because their infection is more likely to be asymptomatic and left untreated for longer.

Hook III and Handsfield (1990) feel that DGI may be missed as a diagnosis because the patient has an asymptomatic genital infection. Pain in the wrists, knees, elbows, ankles or hand joints is common, along with tenosynovitis (Adler, 1990). In some cases one or two large joints are more severely affected and fluid aspirated from the joint is often purulent and will show gonococci (Oates & Csonka, 1990).

About 30% of patients will develop skin lesions. These can be found almost anywhere on the body and initially appear as red papules, which may become pustular and then ulcerated (Oates & Csonka, 1990). They may be present for 5–10 days before healing starts. Hook III and Handsfield (1990) note that patients with gonococcal dermatitis often have arthralgia or tenosynovitis earlier and occasionally disseminated infection may spread to affect the heart or meninges (Adler, 1990). Kundu, Wade and Walzman (1995) note a case of DGI due to penicillinase-producing gonococci, though this is a rare occurrence.

Reiter's syndrome, which is often caused by chlamydia or other non-gonococcal agents, may present with arthritis, genital tract inflammation or conjunctivitis and commonly affects more men than women (Adler, 1990). Oates and Csonka (1990) note that Reiter's syndrome may complicate the diagnosis of DGI. More information about Reiter's syndrome can be found in Chapter 6.

Treatment

Treatment for gonorrhoea depends on various factors but particularly on how effective a particular drug is, the local drug resistance pattern, the cost, the ease of administration, allergic reactions, whether the patient is pregnant and the risk of associated infection (Oates & Csonka, 1990). Hook and Handsfield (1990) note that ideally a single dose treatment should be given to ensure patient compliance, as giving a course of tablets to take away will always result in some patients not finishing the course of treatment or failing to take the correct number of tablets at the correct time.

Some patients are allergic to various antibiotics and patients must always be asked about any allergies before treatment is given. Women should be asked about the risk of pregnancy and the date of the last menstrual period, as some drugs are contraindicated in pregnancy (Oates & Csonka, 1990). It should also be remembered that antibiotics may react with other drugs that the patient is taking.

In the 1930s, sulphonamide drugs were given as treatment until resistance to this group of drugs built up, at which point penicillin became the drug of choice for treatment of gonorrhoea and remained so for many years. By the 1970s penicillin-resistant gonorrhoea was found to be between 18–90% in different parts of the world (Hook III & Handsfield, 1990) and because of this, the World Health Organization (WHO, 1991) recommend the following single dose treatment:

1.   ciprofloxacin 500 mg orally; or
2.   ceftriaxone 250 mg intramuscularly; or
3.   spectinomycin 2 g intramuscularly.

In areas where gonorrhoea is still sensitive to penicillin WHO (1991) suggest the following as single dose therapy:

1.   amoxycillin 3 g with probenecid 1 g orally; or
2.   procaine benzylpenicillin 4.8 million units intramuscularly with probenecid 1 g orally.

Probenecid leads to an increased and prolonged blood level of penicillin (Oates & Csonka, 1990).

The Gonorrhoea Management Standards produced by the National Audit Development Project in Sexual Health (1995) state that in the UK, suitable drugs for treatment of gonorrhoea include ampicillin/amoxycillin either with or without probenecid, ciprofloxacin, ceftriaxone, ceftoxamine, ofloxacin, norfloxacin and spectinomycin, depending on whether the patient is pregnant or allergic to penicillin.

Oates and Csonka (1990) stress that the clinician must know the antibiotic sensitivities in the local gonorrhoea infection as resistance not only varies from place to place but is constantly changing. The National Audit Development Project (1995) note that where a patient has been infected abroad, treatment should be given according to international data on sensitivities.

Drug-resistant gonorrhoea

Tapsall (1995) notes that two mechanisms, chromosomal and extra-chromosomal or plasmid, are involved in the development of antibiotic-resistant gonorrhoea. Plasmid-borne change is normally a one-step process to total resistance, which is how penicillinase-producing *Neisseria gonorrhoea* (PPNG) – also referred to as beta-lactamase producing gonorrhoea – came about. Chromosomal resistance is a slower process, which allows a higher dose of a drug to be given before total resistance occurs (Tapsall, 1995).

PPNG was first recognised in 1976 (Bignell, 1994) and since then has become a major problem in some parts of the world, leading to the use of ceftriaxone, cefoxitin, cefotoxime, spectinomycin, ciprofloxacin and other drugs in the cephalosporin and quinoline groups for treatment of PPNG. In the UK, rates of PPNG have been found to be around 5% between 1982 and 1990 in London (Warren & Phillips, 1993), 5% between 1990 and 1992 in Edinburgh (Ross et al., 1995), but 15% over a one-year period in the early 1990s in a different part of London (Lewis et al., 1995). They also noted that their local population had a high rate of foreign travel, although 96% of their patients with PPNG had been infected in the UK, and the authors had recently changed their drug treatment to ciprofloxacin from amoxycillin with probenecid.

As there are considerable variations in drug resistance worldwide, so clinics are seeing patients with gonorrhoea acquired abroad that is resistant to drugs other than penicillin. Lewis, Forster and Goh (1994) note gonorrhoea resistant to ciprofloxacin coming from Thailand; Thompson, Young and Moyes (1995) note a similar gonorrhoea from Brazil; while Turner et al. (1995) report a gonor-rhoea resistant to penicillin, ciprofloxacin and tetracycline imported from the Philippines.

Such reports confirm Hook III and Handsfield's (1990) belief that the pattern of antibiotic use in a community is the driving force for development of resistance to antibiotics by gonorrhoea infections. It is therefore vitally important that worldwide monitoring of resis-tance patterns is undertaken (Tapsall, 1995).

Epidemiological treatment

Epidemiological treatment is the term used for the treatment of named contacts of patients with gonorrhoea that is given before laboratory results of the tests taken from the contact are available. Physicians often prefer to treat known contacts on an epidemiologi-cal basis, as the patient may default from subsequent appointments that are booked for a time when confirmation of infection is avail-able.

Sherrard and Bingham (1995) believe that epidemiological treat-ment leads to prevalence data being inaccurate nationally. However, the Gonorrhoea Management Standards (National Audit Development Project, 1995) state that epidemiological treatment should be given in the following circumstances:

1.   If the clinician considers the risk of complications from infec-tion to other contacts outweighs the risk of giving the patient unnecessary treatment.
2.   If infection of the cervix, rectum or pharynx is suspected when microscopic diagnosis is relatively unreliable.

The standards highlight the need to undertake confirmatory tests, test of cure and contact tracing even if epidemiological treat-ment is given.

Follow-up procedure

Test of cure is an important part of the control and treatment of gonorrhoea. Sherrard and Bingham (1995) state that patients with gonorrhoea should have one test of cure within 72 hours of treat-ment in case drug resistance causes a persistent infection and a second test of cure about one week after that to treat any postgono-coccal urethritis or chlamydia and exclude reinfection.

Hook III and Handsfield (1990) recommend that all sites known to be infected should be retested and the Gonorrhoea Management Standards (National Audit Development Project, 1995) state that at least one test of cure should be taken, including a rectal sample from all women, as well as other known infected sites, and that a final test of cure should be taken at least 48–72 hours after all antibiotic treatment has finished.

The nurse should emphasise to the patient the need for further tests to ensure the gonorrhoea has been eradicated and also the need for tests to isolate concurrent infections such as trichomoniasis or chlamydia. It is important that the nurse explains to the patient that sexual intercourse should not take place until the patient has been told that the results of the test of cure are negative on culture.

Safer sex

It is the responsibility of the nurse or health adviser who sees the patient to undertake some form of sexual health promotion with all patients attending a GUM department, for whatever reason. The most efficient method of avoiding infection is to use barrier methods of contraception and to have fewer partners. Properly used, condoms have been found to provide a high degree of protection against the transmission of gonorrhoea (Barlow, 1977), as has the diaphragm in the case of cervical infection (Stone, Grimes & Magder, 1986), though the use of spermicides with a diaphragm or condom may also have a role.

Anal intercourse is known to be a high risk behaviour, as rectal mucosa is easily damaged and much more susceptible to infection than the vagina. Therefore, patients should be educated about the risks of anal intercourse, particularly homosexual men who are more likely to undertake this activity. Stone, Grimes and Magder (1986) also suggest that patients should be advised that reducing the number of partners is the most effective way of reducing the risk of being infected with an STD such as gonorrhoea.

Non-specific urethritis

Introduction

Non-specific urethritis (NSU) is a condition resulting in inflammation of the male urethra (urethritis). Following the introduction of Gram staining, it has been possible to differentiate gonococcal from non-gonococcal urethritis (NGU) and many people prefer the term NGU to non-specific urethritis (Csonka, 1990). Both terms will be used in this chapter.

The diagnosis of NSU can be difficult because of its multi-faceted nature and it is often little more than a process of elimination, with possible causes of the condition being examined in detail and a comprehensive history taken from the patient.

Prevalence and transmission

Oriel (1993) notes that up to the 1960s, gonorrhoea was much more common than NSU, but recently gonorrhoea has declined considerably and the incidence of NSU has risen, so that it is now four times that of gonorrhoea and the commonest STD in men in the UK. However, Csonka (1990) believes that the statistics for NGU are not reliable, as many men of a higher social class have NSU and are treated outside GUM clinics. Also NGU is often asymptomatic with recurrences within a year, which may be treated as a new infection rather than a relapse (Csonka, 1990).

NSU is an STD and often cases occur when there is a new sexual partner, with the peak incidence in men aged 20–24 years (Oriel, 1993). Csonka (1990) notes that in comparison with men with gonorrhoea, men with NGU are more likely to be married with a less promiscuous history and from a higher socio-economic group. Men with NGU often have a history of previous NGU infection and although it appears to be transmitted by sexual intercourse, Csonka (1990) believes other host factors play a part, possibly sensitising the man to something in the female partner's genital tract or it is possible that treatment only suppresses the cause of NGU, rather than getting rid of it totally.

McGowan et al. (1991) undertook a small study of men using condoms for safer sex who had NGU and concluded that unprotected oral sex may have had a role in these men developing NGU. It has also been noted that homosexual men are less likely than heterosexual men to have NGU, but more likely to have gonorrhoea (Holmes, 1980).

Carlin and Barton (1995) found that 10% of men seen with NGU had given themselves a variety of treatments, including antibiotics, antiseptic liquid or cream, local anaesthetic gel, vitamins, antifungal cream and even a poultice, before attending GUM. Seventy per cent of the men who had started antibiotics themselves had done so without obtaining a prescription and one man had a drug reaction.

Generally, self-treatment delayed attendance at GUM and affected the results of tests (Carlin & Barton, 1995).

Some patients do not associate the infection with any sexual activity and indeed it may not be related. However, they will attend their general practitioner (GP) complaining of vague symptoms and the GP will often refer these patients directly to the GUM department for accurate diagnosis and treatment. Whatever the cause, symptoms may persist for some time and some patients will present with frequent uncomfortable recurrences of the condition.

Causes of NSU

NSU has many causative agents, not all of them sexually transmitted. It is important therefore that a clear history of events prior to the onset of the symptoms is obtained from the patient, so that the doctor is able to make an accurate diagnosis. The possibility that the urethritis may be caused by an infection that has been sexually acquired or through non-infective means must be properly explained.

The common causes of NSU are shown in Table 5.1. Some are seen much more frequently than others and occasionally there may be several factors related to an episode of NSU.

Table 5.1: Causes of NSU

Chlamydia trachomatis

Ureaplasma urealyticum

Trichomonas vaginalis

Mycoplasma genitalium

Candida albicans?

Haemophilus parainfluenzae?

Corynebacterium genitalium?

Gardnerella vaginalis?

Herpes simplex virus

Urinary tract infections

Allergies

Warts

Foreign bodies

Trauma

Chlamydia trachomatis

Chlamydia is thought to cause 30–50% of all cases of NSU (Csonka, 1990) and is the single most common infection associated with this condition. Holmes (1980) found that only 10–20% of homosexual men with NGU had chlamydia, in comparison to 40% of heterosexual men and that fewer homosexual men than heterosexual men had postgonococcal urethritis caused by chlamydia.

Chlamydia seems to initiate an inflammatory response that may persist even after the infection has been treated with antibiotics and it is possible that an immune mechanism may have a role, thus explaining why chlamydia is found even after treatment (Shahmanesh, 1994).

It is very important that men with NSU are tested for chlamydia, particularly as not only NSU but also chlamydia can be asymptomatic. Further information about chlamydia can be found in Chapter 6.

Ureaplasma urealyticum

Ureaplasma has been found in men with NGU who are chlamydia negative on culture, though it is a difficult organism to type and it is thought that while some strains may be harmless, others may be pathogenic (Csonka, 1990). However, ureaplasma has been found in the majority of sexually active people, with the prevalence increasing with an increase in the number of partners (Shahmanesh, 1994). Therefore, although ureaplasma may cause some cases of NSU, its significance is very uncertain (Oriel, 1993). Viarengo, Hebrant and Piot (1980) found that in a small study of healthy married men, tested weekly for 17 consecutive weeks, 63% had ureaplasma in their urine on at least one occasion, although they could not prove that ureaplasma was a cause of NGU.

In certain cases where ureaplasma has been isolated on culture, it has been necessary to treat both partners to eliminate urethritis (Arya & Pratt, 1986), though this was a small study and may be the exception to the rule.

Other infections causing NSU

Csonka (1990) notes that *Trichomonas vaginalis* (TV) has been seen as a rare cause of NGU. However, unless the urethritis clears quickly after treatment with metronidazole, it is difficult to be sure that the finding of TV is a definite cause of NGU. Oriel (1993) also believes TV only occasionally causes NSU and it is usually asymptomatic in men (Shahmanesh, 1994).

It is possible that *Mycoplasma genitalium* might cause NGU, though this organism is very difficult to culture (Shahmanesh, 1994) and its significance in NGU is uncertain (Csonka, 1990). *Candida albicans* and *Haemophilus parainfluenzae* have also been found in men with NGU, but it is not known if they actually cause it (Csonka, 1990). Oriel (1993) suggests that the *Herpes simplex* virus may also cause NSU through ulceration of the urethra, though not very often. Csonka (1990) suggests that urethritis occurs in up to 40% of cases of herpes but it clears up as the herpes clears. *Corynebacterium genitalium* has been found in 40% of patients with NGU, but also in healthy controls and in men with non-gonococcal epididymitis in an external puncture sample (Csonka, 1990). He also notes that *Gardnerella vaginalis* has been found in 10–20% of the male partners of women with bacterial vaginosis, but the significance of this to urethritis is unclear.

Kumar et al. (1995) investigated the normal urethral flora of young men who had not had sex, in comparison with recently married men with no history of STDs, monogamous patients with NGU and patients with an STD but no urethritis. They found the sexually inactive boys had mostly aerobic flora with a lot of skin flora; in the groups of sexually active men, although aerobes were present, *Staphylococcus aureus* was found much less in the monogamous and inactive boys than in the men with NGU or non-urethritis STDs. Of particular significance was the fact that the isolates from the sexually inactive group were mostly a pure growth but the men in the NGU and STD groups had a mixed growth of organisms and as it is known that following an encounter with vaginal flora, urethral species in men increase, it is believed such newly acquired organisms may have a role in urethral infection (Kumar et al., 1995).

It is believed that NSU may sometimes be part of an upper urinary tract infection (Oriel, 1993). If such infection is suspected, a two-glass urine test should show changes in the second glass of voided urine and a midstream specimen of urine should be sent to the laboratory for culture and sensitivity.

Non-infective causes of NSU

There are thought to be various other causes of NSU. Painting of urethral warts with a solution such as podophyllin may initiate an allergic response (Csonka, 1990), especially if treatment is self-administered. Excessive painting or failure to wash off the paint in the prescribed time may result in damage to the delicate urethral mucosa. The presence of warts within the urethra may cause problems even before treatment is started, depending on their size and position. Treatment of warts by cryotherapy may also result in trauma to the urethra and occasionally post-cryotherapy erosions may lead to urethritis.

It is thought that the overzealous use of disinfectants and antiseptics applied either directly to the penis or added to bath water may have a similar effect to podophyllin in causing NSU, but this is extremely difficult to prove.

Other possible causes include the use of sex toys or aids such as cock rings, which may lead to inflammation and NSU (Csonka, 1990). It is obviously important that patients are asked about such practice, particularly if all other factors have been excluded. It is thought that insertion of foreign bodies into the urethra is more common in homosexual men. Csonka (1990) suggests that some patients indulge in obsessive self-examination with overenthusiastic squeezing of the penis, described as urethrophobia and this in itself may initiate an attack of NSU. Squeezing is often performed by the patient in an attempt to evacuate any possible discharge present.

Postgonococcal urethritis

Adler (1990) suggests that 25–50% of patients with gonorrhoea go on to develop postgonococcal urethritis (PGU) following treatment with penicillin. He suggests that PGU should not be diagnosed until 2 weeks after the original infection has been treated, as it is quite common to find residual urethritis at the first follow-up visit.

Csonka (1990) believes that it can be assumed that patients with PGU are infected with both gonorrhoea and NGU, though Adler (1990) states that in 80% of cases, PGU is caused by chlamydia. There is also a considerable group of patients who have gonococcal urethritis and who develop PGU of unknown cause.

Recurrent or persistent NGU

Oriel (1993) suggests that the cause of recurrent NSU is unknown, but it may be one of the most difficult conditions to manage and Csonka (1990) found it accounted for 10% of the cases of NGU he saw over 5 years.

Various factors may be relevant, such as intercourse with a new partner, resumed intercourse with an untreated partner or non-compliance with treatment (Oriel, 1993). In some cases there may be re-infection; latent infection, particularly in chlamydial infection; or possibly local reactivity (Csonka, 1990). Csonka also notes that some patients get a recurrence of NGU following alcoholic or sexual excess. Oriel (1993) suggests that chronic prostatitis should be considered as a cause of persistent urethritis if all other factors have been eliminated.

It is important that the clinician remains optimistic, as some patients are psychologically affected by persistent or recurrent NGU and overtreatment or overinvestigation can make matters worse (Csonka, 1990; Oriel, 1993).

Clinical features and diagnosis of NGU

The majority of patients will present at a clinic complaining of a urethral discharge and dysuria, though some may only complain of a mild irritation or discomfort at the end of the penis (Csonka, 1990). Up to 20% of patients are found to be completely asymptomatic or to have minimal symptoms (Oriel, 1993) and have attended as a result of contact tracing or for an unrelated problem.

Some patients only see a discharge first thing in the morning before passing urine and these patients may also have urethral discomfort or dysuria first thing (Csonka, 1990). Oriel (1993) notes that in some patients, the end of the penis seems oedematous and congested or there is urethral irritation.

In general, NSU is a much milder disease than gonorrhoea in men, with the symptoms being less severe and often taking longer to appear, if at all. The wide variety of causes means that the incubation period may be anything from a few days to 6 weeks or more, though there is a peak at 2–3 weeks (Csonka, 1990).

Diagnosis is from examination of the urine, normally by the two-glass urine test and by microscopy, backed up by cultures to exclude gonorrhoea and possibly find a causative agent such as chlamydia. The two-glass urine test generally shows specks and threads of pus and white cells in the first glass with the second glass being clear (Csonka, 1990). Oriel (1993) suggests the urine can be centrifuged and the sediment examined as a wet mount, with more than 15 neutrophils per field being diagnostic of urethritis. Dipping the urine with a multistick may show a raised level of leukocytes in the urine, indicating the need for further investigations.

The use of leukocyte esterase (LE) strips has been investigated, particularly for use in countries where access to other tests may be difficult and Tyndall et al. (1994) considered that using LE dipsticks in men with symptomatic urethritis in Kenya improved the accuracy of diagnosis and reduced the amount of antibiotics given without a cause being found. However, Patrick, Rekart and Knowles (1994) felt that in Canada, the use of LE sticks was not a sensitive enough test to accurately diagnose urethritis or urethral pathogens, particularly in asymptomatic men.

Microscopy is done on samples from the urethra and from any discharge. The exact criteria for diagnosis by microscopy may vary, but microscopy should reveal the presence of a large number of polymorphs. Csonka (1990) suggests that some clinicians believe that no leukocytes should be seen in a healthy male, but generally five or more polymorphs seen on several high-power oil immersion fields is taken as diagnostic of NSU (Oriel, 1993), though different clinics may set their own standard diagnostic criteria.

It is important that a careful examination of the slide is undertaken to ensure gonorrhoea is not present. Cultures for gonorrhoea and chlamydia should be taken routinely, regardless of the microscopy findings (Csonka, 1990). If the patient complains of a discharge first thing in the morning only, he may need to attend first thing, without passing urine, for microscopy and urine examination, to allow a diagnosis to be made (Oriel, 1993).

Treatment and management of NSU

The treatment of NSU very much depends on the cause of the urethritis; modifying behaviour may be all that is needed in the case of urethritis of a non-infective nature. Advice may be needed about the use of lotions, etc. that may initiate an allergic response, even if the product has been used for several years without problems. Basic hygiene methods should be discussed and the possibility of urinary tract infections investigated.

Csonka (1990) notes that if NGU is left untreated, it will resolve spontaneously after a few weeks, but it is likely that there will be a recurrence. However, if an infection such as herpes or trichomonas is found correct treatment with aciclovir or metronidazole respectively is recommended (Csonka, 1990).

As the treatment for chlamydia will usually also treat non-chlamydial NSU, the treatment generally used for NSU is either doxycycline 100 mg orally twice a day for 7–14 days or oxytetracycline

500 mg orally four times a day for 7–14 days (Csonka, 1990; Oriel, 1993). If the patient is allergic to tetracycline, then erythromycin 500 mg orally twice daily for 7–14 days can be given. Csonka (1990) also suggests minocycline 100 mg twice daily for 7–14 days or spiramycin 1 g 2–3 times daily for 7 days.

Many researchers feel that it is important to see and treat the female contacts of men with NSU, not only to reduce the chance of reinfection but also because 30% of such female partners are likely to have chlamydia (Oriel, 1993), and Csonka (1990) suggests that 10% of untreated women may develop non-gonococcal PID.

Patients should be seen for follow-up a week after the start of treatment to see whether the treatment has worked, to be given the results of culture tests taken and to check drug compliance (Csonka, 1990). A further appointment should be given for 2 weeks' time to check for signs of persistent or recurrent NGU and for alternative treatment to be given if necessary (Oriel, 1993).

References

Adler MW (1990) ABC of Sexually Transmitted Diseases, 2nd edn. London: British Medical Association.

Andrews H, Acheson N, Huengsberg M, Radcliffe KW (1994) The role of microscopy in the diagnosis of sexually transmitted infections in women. Genitourinary Medicine 70: 118–20.

Arya OP, Pratt BC (1986) Persistent urethritis due to *Ureaplasma urealyticum* in conjugal or stable partnerships. Genitourinary Medicine 62: 329–32.

Barlow D (1977) The condom and gonorrhoea. Lancet October 15: 811–13.

Barlow D, Phillips I (1978) Gonorrhoea in women. Lancet April 8: 761–4.

Bignell C (1994) The eradication of gonorrhoea. British Medical Journal 309: 1103–4.

Carlin EM, Barton SE (1995) How common is self-treatment in non gonococcal urethritis? Genitourinary Medicine 71(6): 400–1.

Csonka GW (1990) Nongonococcal urethritis and postgonococcal urethritis. In Csonka GW, Oates JK (Eds), Sexually Transmitted Diseases – A Textbook of Genitourinary Medicine. London: Baillière Tindall.

DOH (1993) The Health of the Nation: Key Area Handbook HIV/AIDS and Sexual Health. London: HMSO.

Donders GGG, Desmyter J, De Wet DH, Van Assche FA (1993) The association of gonorrhoea and syphilis with premature birth and low birthweight. Genitourinary Medicine 69(2): 98–101.

Edwards S, Dockerty G (1995) Diagnosis of gonorrhoea by microscopy. Genitourinary Medicine 71(3): 200–1.

Evans JK, Mercey DE, French PD, Prince MV (1994) Audit of diagnosis of gonorrhoea at first visit to a London genitourinary medicine clinic. Genitourinary Medicine 70(4): 291–2.

Gutman LT, Wilfert CM (1990) Gonococcal diseases in infants and children. In

Holmes KK, Mårdh P-A, Sparling PF, Wiesner PJ (Eds), Sexually Transmitted Diseases, 2nd edn. New York: McGraw-Hill.

Holmes KK (1980) Nongonococcal urethritis: general considerations and specific considerations for homosexual men. Journal of Homosexuality 5(3): 295–8.

Hook III EW, Handsfield HH (1990) Gonococcal infections in the adult. In Holmes KK, Mårdh P-A, Sparling PF, Wiesner PJ (Eds), Sexually Transmitted Diseases, 2nd edn. New York: McGraw-Hill.

Kinghorn GR, Rashid S (1979) Prevalence of rectal and pharyngeal infection in women with gonorrhoea in Sheffield. British Journal of Venereal Diseases 55: 408–10.

Kumar B, Dawn G, Sharma M, Malla N (1995) Urethral flora in adolescent boys. Genitourinary Medicine 71(5): 328–9.

Kundu A, Wade AAH, Walzman M (1995) Disseminated infection due to penicillin resistant gonococci – is it still rare? Genitourinary Medicine 71(2): 133–4.

Laga M, Plummer FA, Piot P, Datta P, Namaara W, Ndinya-Achola JO, Nzanze H, Maitha G, Ronald AR, Pamba HO, Brunham RC (1988) Prophylaxis of gonococcal and chlamydial ophthalmia neonatorum. New England Journal of Medicine 318(11): 655–7.

Lewis DA, Forster GE, Goh BT (1994) Ciprofloxacin resistant gonococci arriving from Thailand. Genitourinary Medicine 70(5): 360.

Lewis DA, Ison CA, Livermore DM, Chen HY, Hooi AY, Wisdom AR (1995) A one-year survey of *Neisseria gonorrhoeae* isolated from patients attending an east London genitourinary medicine clinic: antibiotic susceptibility patterns and patients' characteristics. Genitourinary Medicine 71(1): 13–17.

Mårdh P-A, Danielsson D (1990) *Neisseria gonorrhoeae*. In Holmes KK, Mårdh P-A, Sparling PF, Wiesner PJ (Eds), Sexually Transmitted Diseases, 2nd edn. New York: McGraw-Hill.

McGowan I, Radcliffe KW, Bingham JS, Dencer C, Ridgway GL (1991) Nongonococcal urethritis in men practising 'safe' sex. Genitourinary Medicine 67(1): 70–1.

National Audit Development Project in Sexual Health (1995) Gonorrhoea management standards. Unpublished.

Oates JK, Csonka GW (1990) Gonorrhoea. In Csonka GW, Oates JK (Eds), Sexually Transmitted Diseases – A Textbook of Genitourinary Medicine. London: Baillière Tindall.

Oriel D (1993) Nonspecific urethritis. Medicine International 21(4):113-15.

Patrick DM, Rekart ML, Knowles L (1994) Unsatisfactory performance of the leukocyte esterase test of first voided urine for rapid diagnosis of urethritis. Genitourinary Medicine 70(3): 187–90.

Ross JDC (1996) Uses and limitations of gonococcal serotyping. International Journal of STD & AIDS 7(1): 14–18.

Ross JDC, Moyes A, McMillan A, Young H (1995) Temporal changes in the sensitivity of *Neisseria gonorrhoeae* to penicillin in Edinburgh, Scotland. International Journal of STD & AIDS 6(2): 110–13.

Ross JDC, Wardropper A, Sprott M, Moyes A, Young H (1994) Gonococcal infection in Edinburgh and Newcastle: serovar prevalence in relation to clinical features and sexual orientation. Genitourinary Medicine 70(1): 35–9.

Shahmanesh M (1994) Problems with non-gonococcal urethritis. International Journal of STD & AIDS 5: 390–9.

THE LIBRARY

KENT & HOSPITAL

TUNBRIDGE WELLS

KENT TN4 8AT

Sherrard JS, Bingham JS (1995) Gonorrhoea now. International Journal of STD & AIDS 6(3): 162–6.

Sparling PF (1990) Biology of *Neisseria gonorrhoeae*. In Holmes KK, Mårdh P-A, Sparling PF, Wiesner PJ (Eds), Sexually Transmitted Diseases, 2nd edn. New York: McGraw-Hill.

Stone KM, Grimes DA, Magder LS (1986) Personal protection against sexually transmitted diseases. American Journal of Obstetrics and Gynecology July: 180–7.

Tapsall JW (1995) Surveillance of antibiotic resistance in *Neisseria gonorrhoeae* and implications for the therapy of gonorrhoea. International Journal of STD & AIDS 6(4): 233–6.

Thin RN, Shaw EJ (1979) Diagnosis of gonorrhoea in women. British Journal of Venereal Diseases 55: 10–13.

Thompson C, Young H, Moyes A (1995) Ciprofloxacin resistant *Neisseria gonorrhoeae*. Genitourinary Medicine 71(6): 412–13.

Turner A, Gough KR, Jephcott AE, McLean AN (1995) Importation into the UK of a strain of *Neisseria gonorrhoeae* resistant to penicillin, ciprofloxacin and tetracycline. Genitourinary Medicine 71(4): 265–6.

Tyndall MW, Nasio J, Maitha G, Ndinya-Achola JO, Plummer FA, Sellors JW, Luinstra KE, Jang D, Mahony JB, Chernesky MA (1994) Leukocyte esterase urine strips for the screening of men with urethritis – use in developing countries. Genitourinary Medicine 70(1): 3–6.

Viarengo J, Hebrant F, Piot P (1980) *Ureaplasma urealyticum* in the urethra of healthy men. British Journal of Venereal Diseases 56: 169–72.

Warren C, Phillips I (1993) Penicillinase producing *Neisseria gonorrhoeae* from St Thomas' Hospital 1976–1990 – the first fifteen years. Genitourinary Medicine 69(3): 210–17.

World Health Organization (1991) Management of patients with sexually transmitted diseases. Geneva: WHO.

Bibliography

Haizlip J, Isbey SF, Hamilton HA, Jeerse AE, Leone PA, Davis RH, Cohen MS (1995) Time required for elimination of *Neisseria gonorrhoeae* from the urogenital tract in men with symptomatic urethritis: comparison of oral and intramuscular single-dose therapy. Sexually Transmitted Diseases May/June:145–8.

McMillan A, Pakianathan M, Mao JH, MacIntyre CCA (1994) Urethral stricture and urethritis in men in Scotland. Genitourinary Medicine 70(6): 403–5.

Schmale JD, Martin (Jr) JE, Domescik G (1969) Observations on the culture diagnosis of gonorrhoea in women. JAMA 210(2): 312–14.

Tice AW, Rodriguez VL (1981) Pharyngeal gonorrhoea. JAMA 246(23): 2717–19.

Chapter 6
Chlamydia and pelvic inflammatory disease

Nicola Church and Alison Sutton

Chlamydia

Introduction

Chlamydia trachomatis infection is recognised as the genital infection responsible for various clinical syndromes in both male and female patients. In males, infection with chlamydia can result in epididymitis, proctitis, conjunctivitis, Reiter's syndrome, non-gonococcal urethritis and postgonococcal urethritis. In females, it can result in Bartholinitis, salpingitis, conjuctivitis, perihepatitis, reactive arthritis and acute urethral syndrome. Over the past 20 years, awareness of the symptoms and the resulting syndromes caused by chlamydia has increased. However, there is still a lot of ignorance among both the general public and the health care professions about the effects of chlamydia, what, if any, the symptoms are and how easily it is passed on.

Recently, there has been media attention focused on people who are experiencing reproductive problems due to infertility caused by chlamydia. This media coverage has done little to explain how chlamydia is passed on or where to go if you feel that you have put yourself at risk. Instead, it has tended to point the finger of blame towards health care professionals for not recognising any symptoms or not giving effective treatment in the early stages. Initially, this caused fear and panic among the public, particularly the female population, but then the subject was dropped from the media and subsequently from general public interest. Therefore, it is important that health care professionals working in genito-urinary medicine (GUM), or any other clinical area, have an understanding of what chlamydia is and its effects so they educate both male and female patients.

Prevalence and risk factors

A high percentage of patients in all clinical settings engage in sexual activity and should therefore be made aware of how chlamydia is passed on and where they can go for a chlamydia test if they feel that they may have been put at risk.

Stamm and Holmes (1990) outline the factors that have led to an increased incidence of chlamydial infections. They argue that it is due to 'inadequate laboratory facilities for their detection and eventual treatment, the nonspecific signs and symptoms chlamydial infections produce, the lack of familiarity clinicians have with these infections, and the lack of resources so far directed toward screening of high-risk patients, contact tracing, and treatment of infected partners'.

Unless a patient visits a GUM clinic, it is highly unlikely that they will be screened for chlamydia: these tests are not normally offered when patients attend their general practitioner (GP) or well person clinic. Some clients believe that when they have a cervical smear taken, this will also detect chlamydia and they therefore see little point in attending a GUM clinic for a check-up.

It has been suggested that the cost of screening for chlamydia may also have contributed to its increased incidence. Some clinicians would not consider testing for chlamydia because of the cost and the inconvenience of testing. The cost of identifying and treating chlamydia by testing urine samples in general practice has been esti- mated to be between £200 and £300 (Dryden et al., 1994). They argue that this is cost effective in comparison with treating the long- term complications of chlamydia in patients and their contacts and that the early detection and treatment of chlamydia will save money in the long term for NHS trusts and GP fundholders. Until the importance of detecting chlamydia is recognised by the government and brought to the forefront of attention through documents such as *The Health of the Nation* (DOH, 1993) – which failed to recognise and mention the increasing rates of chlamydia infection – it will take time for the message to filter through.

The recorded incidence of chlamydia has been assessed mainly in GUM clinics, family planning clinics and antenatal clinics. Some authors have attempted to identify risk groups. Cameron (1993) argues that 'because of its mode of transmission, chlamydial infec- tion most often occurs in the younger sexually active age groups'.

She includes other factors, such as multiple sexual partners, a new partner in the 2 months prior to symptoms arising, attending hospital for a termination of pregnancy, using oral contraception rather than barrier methods of contraception and cervical ectopy or cervicitis, that place a person at risk of infection with chlamydia.

Although Cameron (1993) outlines these groups as at risk, it must be remembered that any person who is sexually active is at risk. It has been stated by Hammerschlag, Handsfield and Judson (1987) that up to 80% of women and 10–20% of men can be asymptomatic. This should be remembered when taking a client's sexual history and assessing if they should be screened. Even if they do not fit into the 'at risk' categories and are asymptomatic, they could still have a positive result.

Biology of chlamydia

Chlamydiae are microorganisms classified as bacteria, that have the characteristics of both bacteria and viruses. *Chlamydia trachomatis* is one of the two species within the genus that are of concern. It is specific only to humans and has, in total, 15 serotypes: types A, B, Ba and C, which cause eye infections; types D to K, which are responsible for genital infections but can affect the eyes, if the organism is transmitted from the genital tract; and finally L1, L2 and L3, which cause lymphogranuloma venereum.

The other species in the genus, *Chlamydia psittaci*, is a common pathogen in birds and domestic mammals and can be passed on to humans who are in close contact with them. The result in humans is a pneumonitis with moderate to severe systemic symptoms. It has been found to be common in the elderly, who often keep birds in their living rooms.

Chlamydiae rely on host cells for energy, as do viruses. They are restricted to an intracellular lifestyle because they lack the ability to synthesise high energy compounds and depend on the host cell to supply them with any necessary nutrients. Schachter (1990) describes chlamydia as an 'intracellular parasite'. The growth cycle initially involves attachment to and then penetration of a susceptible host cell; it then remains in a phagocytic vesicle throughout the rest of the growth cycle. Following the initial attachment and entry into the cell, morphologic change to the reticulate body with intracellular growth and replication takes place. There is then a further morphologic change to the elementary body, before the infectious particles are released. The host cell dies following this release. The whole growth cycle takes between 48 and 72 hours to complete. There is then an incubation period of between 7 and 21 days before symptoms appear, if any do. The patient can remain asymptomatic for years until the infection has developed into an associated syndrome.

Clinical features in men

In men, chlamydial urethral infection usually presents with the symptoms of a non-specific urethritis. The patient will have a discharge from the urethra, which can be either mucopurulent or thin and watery. He may suffer pain or discomfort when passing urine. He could also be completely asymptomatic and be presenting for testing because of a contact he has had. On genital examination, the male usually reveals no other problems apart from discharge. Abnormal prostatic examinations have not been strongly linked to chlamydial urethritis. It has been well documented that chlamydia is more often asymptomatic than gonococcal urethral infection and when symptoms do occur they are milder with chlamydial urethritis.

Berger et al. (1978) have shown that chlamydia causes most cases of what was previously termed idiopathic epididymitis, in young sexually active males. Chlamydial epididymitis presents as unilateral scrotal pain, swelling, tenderness and fever in a man who has had an associated chlamydial urethritis. Epididymitis is treated with a form of tetracycline for a period of up to 2 weeks.

Despite the continued study, the role of chlamydia in causing non-bacterial prostatitis remains controversial. Studies that support the claim that chlamydia causes prostatitis have been conducted, while others question this claim. Poletti et al. (1985) performed transrectal biopsies of the prostate on 30 men who had a known positive chlamydia urethral culture and a diagnosis of non-bacterial prostatitis, which was based on prostatic tenderness or swelling upon digital palpation. Of the 30 men, the organism was isolated in 10 of their prostatic specimens, which suggests that chlamydia may have a role in non-bacterial prostatitis. Nilsson, Johannisson and Lycke (1981) reported a recovery of chlamydia from the expressed prostatic secretions of 26 men who all had acute non-gonococcal urethritis. Taken together, the work on whether chlamydia causes prostatitis is still unclear. However, it is well documented that there is a link.

Reiter's syndrome

Keat and Rowe (1990) argue that sexually transmitted genital infection is probably the major cause of inflammatory arthritis in young adults in the Western world. Approximately one third of patients with reactive arthritis, irrespective of the type of initiating infection, have the characteristic features of Reiter's syndrome, which are: peripheral arthritis, genital tract inflammation and ocular inflammation. The essential feature of Reiter's syndrome is the relationship between an infection at one site and aseptic inflammation at another. It is believed that synovitis and possibly other lesions result from the action of mediators released into the circulation which are eventually deposited within the synovium, where the process of inflammation begins (Keat & Rowe, 1990). Reiter's syndrome is regarded as a predominantly male syndrome.

Reiter's syndrome is now linked with both gonococcal and non-gonococcal urethritis. Attempts to isolate chlamydia from the synovium and synovial fluid have been hampered by clinical and technical difficulties but have been almost universally negative. Keat et al. (1987) demonstrated the presence of chlamydial elementary bodies in the synovium of five out of eight patients with sexually acquired reactive arthritis (SARA) and all five patients also had high titres of specific chlamydial antibody in their serum. This suggests that there is a strong link between SARA and chlamydia.

Attempts to isolate chlamydia from the eye have almost always proved negative. Dawson et al. (1970) were able to demonstrate eye involvement in 13 out of 24 patients with Reiter's syndrome, who also had evidence of chlamydial infection. Few other examples appear to have been documented.

Not all patients with Reiter's syndrome present with urethral chlamydia. Around 10% of patients who present with SARA have gonorrhoea (Keat & Rowe, 1990). Gonococcal antigens in the joint are known to induce arthritis experimentally. At the moment, the role that gonorrhoea plays has to be resolved, though it is probably significant.

The clinical features of Reiter's syndrome are described as follows. Dysuria or urethral discharge is frequently the first symptom; joint symptoms may occur at the same time or following the urethral symptoms. Synovitis normally develops within 30 days of the onset of symptoms of infection in 90% of patients (Keat & Rowe, 1990). The initial joints involved are usually the knee, ankle or metatarso-phalangeal joints. New joints become involved usually over a period of 2 to 3 weeks. Up to 10% of patients have a persistent monoarthritis and many of the remainder develop oligoarticular or disease in two to five joints.

Lesions on the mucus membranes and the skin can occur in patients with Reiter's syndrome, particularly on the feet and genital area. Uveitis can also occur during an attack of arthritis. It is difficult to distinguish from conjuctivitis and appears as a painful red eye, but it is important to distinguish the difference as it can infrequently lead to corneal ulceration, intraocular haemorrhage or optic neuritis (Keat & Rowe, 1990).

After a period of 3 to 5 months following the initial attack, the synovitis normally starts to subside. The symptoms can last for up to a year and can come back over several years. The prognosis for the majority of patients is good. It is recognised that females go undetected for a long period of time because their cervical infection with chlamydia can be asymptomatic.

Infertility

Much attention has been drawn to female infertility caused by chlamydia, but little attention has been directed at male fertility and whether it is affected by chlamydia. Greendale et al. (1993) looked at the relationship between chlamydia and unexplained infertility in men. They took serum from 52 men who were infertile and 79 men who were first time expectant fathers. They also gave them a detailed questionnaire to fill in. In conclusion, Greendale et al. (1993) found that their results suggested an association between chlamydia and unexplained male infertility and implied that this was due to asymptomatic infection with chlamydia. Further work in this area is needed to perhaps offer an explanation for male infertility.

Clinical features in women

Although many women with chlamydia isolated from the cervix have no signs or symptoms of infection, many do have localised signs. Most commonly observed is a mucopurulent discharge, which can be found on a speculum examination. Hypertrophic ectopy of the cervix is also a common localised symptom with the ectopy being oedematous, congested and bleeding easily when touched with a swab. Harrison et al. (1985) argue that the prevalence of chlamydial infection appears greater in women with ectopy than in those without ectopy. The ectopy may expose a greater number of susceptible columnar epithelial cells, making infection more likely, or it may increase the shedding of chlamydia from the cervix. Stamm and Holmes (1990) suggest that this is the reason why chlamydia is found in the younger age groups. Cervical ectopy is normally found to be present in 60–80% of sexually active adolescents and then declines when women are in their thirties and forties. A Gram stain of endocervical discharge from a patient with endocervicitis usually shows more than 30 pus cells per 1000 field. This can also be used as a marker when trying to make a diagnosis.

Urethritis due to chlamydia often goes undetected due to lack of symptoms from the urethra. It has been widely documented that symptoms of dysuria and frequency occur in women with chlamydia urethritis, but it can be asymptomatic.

Chlamydia has also been linked to purulent infections of Bartholin's ducts causing Bartholinitis. This is a localised inflammation of the Bartholin's duct, which is painful to touch.

If chlamydia remains untreated, it may spread through the uterus into the fallopian tubes where acute salpingitis can cause scarring, which in turn blocks the tubes and may eventually cause infertility. Both salpingitis and endometritis are discussed in further detail in this chapter under the heading of Pelvic Inflammatory Disease (PID).

Clinical features in neonates

Another group who are at risk of developing chlamydia are babies born to mothers who have chlamydia during pregnancy. There is speculation that pregnancy influences the amount of shedding of chlamydia. Brunham, Holmes and Embree (1990) suggest that two thirds of neonates become infected with chlamydia in the eyes when in the birth canal. Infants who are born to mothers who have chlamydia, or who have had a previous chlamydial infection, acquire antibodies to this organism. The influence of these antibodies on the risk of acquisition is not known. The presence of chlamydia antibodies in breast milk or colostrum has not been documented as having any influence in preventing or modifying neonatal chlamydial infection. It should, therefore, be pointed out to pregnant women who have chlamydia that there is a risk of the babies developing ocular chlamydia. Infants born to infected mothers will develop conjunctivitis between the first and third weeks following delivery.

The symptoms are a mucopurulent unilateral or bilateral eye discharge accompanied with a red, sore eye. Whelan (1988) states that some infants will go on to develop chlamydia pneumonia, which will manifest itself between 1 and 3 months of age. Postnatal care of the mother and baby should include regular follow-up appointments for up to 3 months because of this risk.

Testing

To ensure accurate detection of chlamydia the specimen for testing must be appropriately collected and transported. The collection of such a specimen is outlined in chapter 1.

When testing for chlamydia, cell culture is considered to be the gold standard test, accurately diagnosing 60% of positive chlamydia samples, though Ridgway and Taylor-Robinson (1992) outline this method as both expensive and time consuming. It involves the use of McCoy cells, which are treated with cycloheximide, with one blind passage and staining of the cell mondayer with a monoclonal immunofluorescent antibody. This method of cell culture is still regarded by many as the method of choice for the most accurate diagnosis. However, it is thought to be far from perfect. The destruction of cells while specimens are being handled is a problem. However, the high specificity of the cell culture in competent hands is trusted by many physicians, and other methods of testing are considered to be inferior.

Smears taken from the urethra and the cervix can be fixed and stained and then analysed for the chlamydia organism. This technique is no longer widely used because of problems with processing the sample in the laboratory. The smear is first air-dried and then stained in the laboratory. In order to detect a chlamydia cell a member of the laboratory staff has to read the slide in a darkened room. If there are many slides to read, staff resources can be a problem and this increases the chance of human error. Another problem appears to be that some patients who have a positive chlamydia on smear, then go on to have a negative culture result. It would seem that more work is needed to analyse this discrepancy.

In contrast to using vital dyes, the use of fluorescein-conjugated monoclonal antibodies is far more successful. Taylor-Robinson (1992) argues that the use of direct fluorescent antibody (DFA) tests has definitely made an impact on the diagnosis of chlamydia over the last few years. As in the use of vital dyes, DFA tests stain the whole inclusions in cells, and have been used predominantly to stain extra-cellular chlamydial elementary bodies in ocular and genital smears. The sensitivity of this test ranges from 70–100% in men and from 68–100% in women. It has been shown to have both good sensitivity and specificity when used by staff who are able to detect small numbers of less than 10 elementary bodies with confidence. The accuracy of DFA tests is still largely dependent on the skill and expertise of the laboratory staff in interpreting the results.

Over the past couple of years various enzyme immunoassays have been introduced. The reading of these tests is neither subjective nor tedious and they can be processed by a machine which will also produce a final report following the testing. The problem with this method is that it is insensitive, like the DFA test. Taylor-Robinson (1992) looked at sensitivity values and argued that this test is 62–97% sensitive in men and 64–98% in women. A positive result should, therefore, be confirmed by testing the remains of the transport medium by immunofluorescence with a specific monoclonal antibody or by using a specific blocking antibody. It is impossible to check all negative results using this method and it is difficult to detect any false negative results.

At the moment there is a lot of interest in the development of the polymerase chain reaction (PCR) as a method of testing. This type of test aims to improve the sensitivity and therefore improve the reliability of this test. Mahony et al. (1990) consider PCR to be slightly less sensitive than the gold standard of cell culture testing. Others have found that this test has a high specificity and sensitivity. The PCR method is not widely used at the moment, but following further development, PCR will probably be the test universally used in GUM clinics in future.

There has been a lot of work carried out in the area of sampling. There is much debate as to whether or not urethral swabs taken for chlamydia are as effective as the first catch of urine (FCU) when trying to detect chlamydia using the enzyme immunoassay (EIA) method of testing. Kok et al. (1993) studied two groups of patients to determine whether the use of urine samples from male patients could replace urethral swabs for the rapid detection of chlamydia by EIA. They found that when EIA was validated against cell culture, it showed a sensitivity of 100% and a specificity of 95% for a swab taken from the urethra. In comparison, the urine specimens were positive in 24% of patients who yielded a positive result on the urethral swab. They concluded therefore that the use of urine samples could not replace urethral swabs for the laboratory diagnosis of chlamydia. However, Patel et al. (1991) in their study found that in urine sampling, 94% of samples came back positive and on urethral swabs only 72% came back positive. Crowley et al. (1992) also support the argument that an FCU sample is a sensitive method and has the advantage of being non-invasive. In their study they compared the effectiveness of first catch early morning urine samples against urethral swabs and found that 91% of cases detected chlamydia from the FCU and only 65% from urethral swabs. The study also shows that flushing the urethra by voiding urine does not appear to affect the detection of chlamydia from urethral swabs.

Hay et al. (1993) compared the detection rates of chlamydia from first pass urine samples tested by an amplified enzyme-linked immunosorbent assay (ELISA) and the detection rates from urethral samples tested by DFA tests. Their results concluded that the sensitivity of using the FCU samples was 90% and the sensitivity of the direct fluorescent antibody test was 83%. They also concluded that the adoption of testing FCU samples for chlamydia would not lead to a decrease in sensitivity in detecting chlamydia and would be more acceptable to patients than urethral swabbing.

Although the use of a urine specimen to detect chlamydia in men is an attractive alternative to the use of the urethral swab and has been proven to be as effective as both ELISA and DFA tests, the urethral culture for chlamydia remains the test of preference among physicians up and down the country. Kok et al. (1993) contend that in order for urine specimens to replace male urethral swabs, the urine test sensitivity would need to be 95% when compared with the urethral positive specimens tested in the same system. They suggest that the use of different assays in other laboratories may account for the varying sensitivities reported in other studies.

Urine sampling in female attenders is considered to be of little value. Patel et al. (1991) sampled 455 women and found that urethral carriage of chlamydia is infrequent compared with that of the endocervix. It is argued that cleaning the vulva before taking the tests, which is common practice, can alter the sensitivity of the swab taken from the urethra. Therefore, it is not considered suitable to take a swab for chlamydia from the urethra of females.

It can be seen that the majority of the authors mentioned are in favour of the use of FCU samples tested by EIA or ELISA for the detection of chlamydia. The suggestion that this form of testing is more patient-friendly can have further implications when considering the attendance rates of clinics and compliance with treatment.

Treatment

Once chlamydia has been isolated, treatment in this initial stage is paramount, before it goes on to develop into anything more serious, such as PID. Chlamydia can be treated with antibiotics such as doxycycline or erythromycin and as it produces folic acid, chlamydia is also sensitive to the action of sulphonamides and to trimethoprim. Sulphonamides have been clinically effective in the treatment of trachoma and lymphogranuloma venereum, but are not used in treating most genital tract infections. Tetracyclines and erythromycin are generally considered the drugs of choice in managing chlamydial genital tract infections (Schachter, 1990). Resistance to these drugs has not been shown to occur naturally, although there are documented treatment failures where chlamydia has been isolated from patients following treatment. Chlamydia does have a bacteria-like cell wall and its synthesis can be inhibited by penicillins, but only in the early phases of the growth cycle, which is why penicillins are not used in the treatment of chlamydia.

For the treatment of uncomplicated urethral, endocervical or rectal chlamydia infections in adults, Whelan (1988) recommends a tetracycline-based drug 500 mg four times a day for 7 days or doxycycline 500 mg twice a day for 7 days. Erythromycin is considered to be the drug of choice if a patient is pregnant and a dose of 500 mg four times a day is recommended. If a patient is unable to tolerate such a high dose, then a lower dose over a longer period of time is recommended. Each GUM clinic has its own protocol for the treatment of uncomplicated chlamydia. In cases of epididymo-orchitis, dual therapy for chlamydia and gonorrhoea is recommended, as is also the case with PID.

Some researchers have suggested treating patients for both gonorrhoea and chlamydia at the same time. Stamm et al. (1984) argued that 15% of men and 26% of women treated for gonorrhoea in their study were also positive for chlamydia and therefore treatment for gonorrhoea should also be effective against chlamydia. They found that tetracycline was effective against both gonorrhoea and chlamydia in men, as was trimethoprim-sulfamethoxazole, and both were well tolerated and reasonably priced. However, in women the effective treatment for gonorrhoea and chlamydia of trimethoprim-sulfamethoxazole was more expensive and caused 36% of the women to have neurological side effects which, though reversible, could reduce compliance (Stamm et al., 1984). There is also the problem of how patients feel about being treated for two infections and whether this could cause extra problems in their relationships.

Neonatal inclusion conjunctivitis or afebrile pneumonia can be treated with erythromycin. A dose of 50 mg per kg of body weight four times a day for 14 days is currently recommended. The child may require a hospital admission until the treatment regimen is established and any side effects have been observed. Brunham, Holmes and Embree (1990) suggest that pregnant women should be treated with erythromycin 400 mg four times a day for 7 days.

Higher daily doses of erythromycin are not well tolerated by pregnant women in the first trimester of pregnancy and this should be borne in mind when deciding on treatment regimens.

Follow-up care

Following treatment, all patients should be followed up and the test for chlamydia repeated to try and assess if the treatment has been successful. Any sexual contacts of the infected patient should also be screened and given treatment to prevent the infection being passed backwards and forwards between the partner(s) and anyone else.

If the patient has been tested in a GUM clinic and has a positive result, then an attempt will be made to trace the patient's contact or contacts. This service is often omitted in other specialities and by GPs, but can be vital in the prevention of re-infection of the patient and the overall spread of the disease. The procedure of contact tracing is described in Chapter 3.

It is difficult to over-emphasise the importance of contact tracing in chlamydia infection. As stated earlier, both men and women can be asymptomatic and not feel the need to attend the clinic for a check up. Cameron (1993) suggests that men and women diagnosed through contact tracing are usually asymptomatic, which can lead to more serious problems for them in the future. To improve contact tracing and thus ensure the incidence of chlamydia and associated syndromes decreases, greater cooperation between specialities, such as obstetrics and gynaecology and urology, is needed.

Conclusion

In conclusion, the effects of *Chlamydia trachomatis* both physically and emotionally can be immense. To prevent the further spread of disease, education of health care professionals and the general public should be at the forefront of any sexual health programme – in schools of medicine, nursing, general educational institutions and in media campaigns.

The availability of chlamydia screening should also be increased and it should be included as part of the panel of diagnostic tests taken when a doctor is trying to establish a diagnosis from symptoms expressed by the patient.

The inclusion of all specialities in the programme of contact tracing should also be considered to try and reduce re-infection and further decrease transmission. It has been suggested that a greater effort is needed by all health care professionals to recognise patients at risk, symptoms, if there are any, and how and where to obtain a chlamydia test. Unless the problem of the increased incidence of chlamydia and its effects are recognised, there will be more cases of infertility in both males and females. This will make the headlines and may cause great emotional pain to childless couples.

Pelvic inflammatory disease

Introduction

Pelvic inflammatory disease (PID) is generally defined as inflammation of the upper genital tract (Hare, 1990a). MacLean (1995) describes pelvic infection as 'infection of the uterus, uterine tubes, adjacent parametria and overlying pelvic peritoneum', and goes on to use the term PID to describe the clinical features of sexually transmitted pelvic infections affecting women of childbearing age. The organs involved therefore, are the uterus, fallopian tubes, ovaries and the tissue surrounding them, often the pelvic peritoneum. PID is usually caused by ascending infection from the cervix, generally bacterial, which causes pelvic infection. Weström and Mårdh (1990) also include pelvic (tubal and tubo-ovarian) abscess in their definition of PID. Hare (1990b) notes that some authors use the term salpingitis and others use PID, however the term PID will be used in this chapter.

Causative agents

There are many microorganisms that have been shown to cause PID. Pelvic infection was noted over 100 years ago and was originally thought to be of tuberculous and non-tuberculous origin. Some authors divide PID into gonococcal and non-gonococcal infections (MacLean, 1995). However, following an increase in PID associated with chlamydia, other researchers have divided causative agents into sexually transmitted or exogenous agents and those organisms that live naturally in the lower genital tract or endogenous agents (Weström & Mårdh, 1990).

The number of new cases of pelvic infection seen in GUM clinics in England has risen from 4 954 in 1989 to 7 690 in 1994 (DOH, 1995). It is interesting to note that of the new cases of pelvic infection seen in GUM in 1994, the vast majority, 6 949, were found to be of non-specific origin, that is no causative agent was traced. Eighty-nine gonococcal, 575 chlamydial and 77 mixed gonococcal and chlamydial cases of pelvic infection were diagnosed in 1994. Weström and Mårdh (1990) note that 'the multitude of species in the lower genital tract of all women as well as the inaccessibility of the fallopian tubes for sampling have long been major obstacles in studies of the etiology of PID'. The problems of diagnosing PID from cervical and vaginal specimens will be discussed later.

Neisseria gonorrhoea produces a classic gonococcal PID, described by many authors from early this century to modern times. Before antibiotics were used this gonococcal PID was generally self-limiting, and lasted 10–14 days unless secondary infection occurred (Hare, 1990a). The incubation time for gonorrhoea infection is 2–14 days and most men infected with gonorrhoea will have symptoms. However, 60% of women with gonorrhoea will be asymptomatic, though some women may go on to develop arthritis, dermatitis, gonococcal septicaemia or PID. MacLean (1995) suggests that some of the tubal damage from gonorrhoea is due to toxin released by the organism, which reduces the activity of the cilia lining the tubes.

It appears that the prevalence of gonococcal PID is falling in Europe, though not elsewhere in the world (Hare, 1990a), but the reason for this is not clear. Also, researchers have found that many patients who have gonorrhoea on the cervix and active PID do not have gonorrhoea in tubal specimens. It is believed that gonorrhoea may be overgrown and replaced by other secondary organisms leading to a multiple pathology (MacLean, 1995). Overall, gonorrhoea should be suspected in cases of PID especially in young, sexually active women.

Chlamydia trachomatis was first isolated in fallopian tubes in 1976 (Hare, 1990a) and it has now been established as an important pathogen in cases of acute and chronic PID (Weström & Mårdh, 1990). MacLean (1995) states that chlamydia is now the most common sexually transmitted organism in the UK and possibly throughout the Western world. It appears that the ratio of chlamydia- to gonorrhoea-linked PID is increasing in Europe (Weström & Mårdh, 1990). In women with PID who undergo laparoscopy, chlamydia has been isolated from tubal specimens in over 30% of cases. Additionally, women having a diagnostic laparoscopy to investigate infertility have been found to have chlamydia infection in their fallopian tubes and chlamydia antibodies in serum on blood test, showing evidence of previous chlamydial infection, frequently undiagnosed.

It is believed that chlamydial PID tends to be milder in clinical severity than gonococcal PID but can be more of a long-term problem.

It has been found that, as with gonorrhoea, chlamydia can be over-grown and other non-sexually transmitted infections may cause a rapid exacerbation of symptoms that often leads the patient to seek medical help (Hare, 1990a).

Mycoplasma and ureaplasma organisms have been found to be a cause of PID and pelvic abscess formation (Hare, 1990a), though the role of these organisms as upper genital tract pathogens is unclear. Weström and Mårdh (1990) note that *Mycoplasma hominis* has not been isolated from macroscopically normal tubes but is frequently isolated from the cervix and vagina of women without signs or symptoms of cervicitis or PID. Mycoplasmas and ureaplasmas are also thought to contribute to non-specific urethritis in men (MacLean, 1995). It has been noted that antibodies to these organisms have been found in women demonstrated to have PID. However, Hare (1990b) notes that the very high rates of isolation of mycoplasmas and ureaplasmas from healthy women make it extremely difficult to find out whether these organisms are acting as pathogens, opportunistic pathogens or just incidental colonisers. These organisms are treated with tetracycline and related drugs that are also used to treat chlamydia, so it is likely that possible infection caused by them will be dealt with adequately. Weström and Mårdh (1990) comment on the fact that many patients appear to have more than one STD pathogen isolated in acute PID and suggest that cultures from the upper genital tract might help the study of the role of different STD agents in PID.

Endogenous aerobic and anaerobic bacteria are found in women with bacterial vaginosis and Hare (1990b) notes that many authors have reported isolating such organisms from severe cases of PID, especially where there is abscess formation. Weström and Mårdh (1990) include the following organisms as having been found in the upper genital tract: facultative and anaerobic streptococci, including group B streptococci and peptostreptococci; *Escherichia coli*; *Gardnerella vaginalis*; *Bacteroides* species, especially *B. melaninogenicus* and *B. bivius*; and clostridial and actinomyces species. They also note that polymicrobial infection has often been demonstrated by culture of specimens obtained by laparoscopy, but where cultures have been obtained by culdocentesis or transcervical endometrial aspiration, results should be interpreted with caution because of the risk of contamination of such specimens with vaginal bacteria. Hare (1990b) suggests that it is possible that anaerobic organisms may cause infection to develop in women whose fallopian tubes have previously been damaged by chlamydia or gonorrhoea.

Viruses are thought to have a role in PID, though there have not been many attempts at isolating viruses from women with PID (Weström & Mårdh, 1990). They suggest that further studies should be done on the possible role of viral infections in the upper genital tract. Hare (1990a) notes that the isolation of *Herpes simplex* in the tubes or endometrium of a few women with observed acute salpingitis and herpetic lesions of the lower genital tract, seems to suggest that herpetic PID is a possibility.

Miscellaneous agents, such as respiratory tract and mouth organisms, have been found in women with PID and Hare (1990a) suggests that orogenital sexual practices, such as the blowing of air into the vagina, may possibly lead to the upward spread of organisms present in the genital area or passed on from the sexual partner's mouth. Weström and Mårdh (1990) also note that in a few cases, tropical disease organisms have been found in PID but these are thought to be rare. In many cases of PID no causative agent is found, though there is definite evidence of salpingitis.

Risk factors

There are various risk factors that may contribute to the development of PID. Weström and Mårdh (1990) note that the risk of acquiring PID seems to decrease with the increasing age of sexually experienced women. MacLean (1995) notes that PID is never found in girls before puberty and very rarely in women after the menopause. Rome (1994) says that adolescents continue to be the age group at highest risk of being infected with an STD and developing PID. Weström and Mårdh (1990) feel that there is no proven explanation why girls between the ages of 15 and 24 are at such risk of PID. However, these authors all feel that the low levels of protective antibodies in the local immune system from lack of previous exposure to pathogens, cervical ectopy, the changes in the functional cervical barrier and the high prevalence of gonorrhoea and chlamydia in this age group might be important factors.

It appears that the risk of PID is definitely linked to sexual activity. MacLean (1995) notes that virginal women rarely have PID and it is much more likely in those who have multiple partners. PID is only seen in sexually active women and Weström and Mårdh (1990) state that the relationship between sexual activity and the risk of PID is valid even if the PID is not associated with chlamydial or gonococcal infection.

In addition, it has been noted by many authors that the use of intrauterine devices (IUDs) may give up to a 10-fold increase in the risk of developing PID. It has been observed that PID tends to occur in IUD-users within 4 months of insertion of the device. It has also been suggested that many IUD-users have chronic endometritis and endosalpingitis (Wølner-Hanssen, Kiviat & Holmes, 1990). Rome (1994) advised that 'adolescents who often have multiple partners, serial monogamy, and more frequent exposure to STDs are generally not good candidates for IUDs'.

PID can also follow surgical procedures such as termination of pregnancy, dilatation and curettage, and tubal insufflation, as well as following miscarriage (spontaneous abortion) and childbirth.

Disease spread

Various factors are thought to be relevant to how infection spreads from the lower genital tract to cause PID. It appears that sperm on their natural progression to the fallopian tubes for fertilisation may act as a vector for infection (Hare, 1990a). The female partners of men with low sperm counts or who are azoospermic have much less risk of PID.

It has also been noted that the 'in-suck' phenomenon during intercourse, when pressure changes in the uterus cause material to be sucked into it from the vagina, may have a role in the spread of pathogens causing PID.

During menstruation, blood can flow in a retrograde fashion from the uterus up the tubes, and Weström and Mårdh (1990) note that microorganisms might spread with such blood, contributing to the development of PID. Once infection has spread to the uterus causing endometritis, the only things that stop the spread of infection to the fallopian tubes are the small size of the tubal openings in the uterus and the flow of mucus, helped by the tubal cilia, from the tubes to the uterus.

Hare (1990a) summarises by describing PID in the following way:

• Primary PID: an infection which occurs usually in a young woman with no previous damage to the upper genital tract and where some form of transport mechanism is needed for the organism to penetrate the cervical barrier. These infections are often started by STD agents, though inflamed tissues may later be colonised by normal bowel and vaginal organisms.

• Secondary PID: this normally occurs when the barrier has been breached or damaged in some way, by surgery, childbirth, miscarriage or pregnancy for example. These infections are more often caused by aerobic and anaerobic organisms than primary PID.

• Recurrent PID: a previous infection means a woman is at high risk of recurrent infection often by non-STD organisms. However, there is no definite link between clinical presentation and the type of organism causing infection.

The process of pelvic infection has been described as either acute or chronic by various authors. Acute infection is normally bilateral though the tubes may look different (MacLean, 1995). Macroscopically, the fallopian tubes are swollen and reddened on the outside surface, though at the open fimbriated ends the tubal mucosa is normally congested and very red and exudate can be seen coming from the tubes (Weström & Mårdh, 1990). Microscopically or on histology, the inflammatory process causes oedema of the tubal mucosa and serous exudate fills the lumen, often causing folds of the mucosa to stick to each other (Weström & Mårdh, 1990; MacLean, 1995).

As the infection gets more severe, the inflammation increases and the tubes are less freely movable, and are often stuck to nearby pelvic structures. In chronic PID, the tubes are usually very distorted with extensive dilatation and often with formation of a hydrosalpinx (fluid filled tube) or pyosalpinx (pus-filled tube). The tubes may become thickened and obstructed (MacLean, 1995). Weström and Mårdh (1990) note that at this stage the whole pelvic cavity can be filled by an inflammatory mass in which it is difficult to see the various structures. Often tubal or tubo-ovarian abscesses form and these may involve loops of bowel. Figure 6.1 shows the swollen fallopian tube seen in PID.

Diagnosis

A diagnosis of PID can be extremely difficult to make. Hare (1990b) noted that 'the accuracy of clinical diagnosis of lower abdominal pain in a woman of childbearing age is low'. Stacey and Munday (1994) comment that this difficulty of diagnosis in lower abdominal pain is because the signs and symptoms are often vague and pain may resolve and recur without any specific treatment and without a definite diagnosis being made. Acute PID can vary clinically from an asymptomatic to a life-threatening condition, though often the

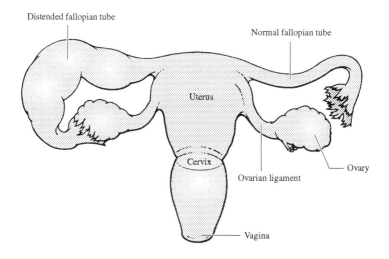

Figure 6.1: Swollen fallopian tube

patient is not seriously ill with gonococcal or chlamydial PID (Weström & Mårdh, 1990).

Diagnosis of PID is also affected by the fact that so many microbial species are normal in the lower genital tract of women and also that it is difficult to sample from the upper genital tract without some form of surgical procedure. MacLean (1995) notes that the frequent lack of microbial support is very frustrating when diagnosing recurrent or chronic PID. Commonly there are differences in what is isolated from the upper and lower genital tracts in PID (Weström & Mårdh, 1990). This is partly explained by the fact that both chlamydia and gonorrhoea can be overgrown, allowing endogenous infections to colonise instead.

These lower genital tract infections may have been asymptomatic or caused only mild and short-lived symptoms preceding the PID. It is possible for the lower genital tract infection to have been present for months before PID complicates the issue (Weström & Mårdh, 1990). Hare (1990a) notes that once a diagnosis of PID has been made, it tends to persist as a label, with further episodes of pain being diagnosed as recurrent PID without alternatives being much considered, even when the original diagnosis was made because no other cause was found.

This difficulty of diagnosis means that rigid criteria for clinical diagnosis are necessary. Hager et al. (1983) looked at the problems of diagnosing PID and suggested rigid criteria for clinical diagnosis, as shown in Table 6.1.

Table 6.1: Clinical criteria for diagnosis and grading of salpingitis
(Hager et al., 1983)

All of the following are required for the diagnosis of salpingitis:
1. Abdominal tenderness when the patient is palpated, rebound may or may not be present.
2. When moving the cervix and uterus, there is excitation tenderness.
3. Bi-manual palpation reveals adnexal tenderness.

One or more of the following are also required:
4. Gram stain of the endocervix positive for Gram-negative intracellular diplococci.
5. Temperature higher than 38 °C.
6. A white cell count of more than 10 000 WBC/mm.
7. Pus-stained fluid containing white cells obtained from the peritoneal cavity when culdocentesis or laparoscopy is performed.
8. On bi-manual examination or by ultrasound, a pelvic abscess or inflammation is detected.

The following stages are suggested when clinical examination is performed:
I. Uncomplicated or limited to tubes and/or ovaries. Pelvic peritonitis may or may not be present.
II. Complicated, when an inflammatory mass or tubal or tubo-ovarian abscess is present and pelvic peritonitis may or may not be present.
III. Structures beyond the pelvis involved e.g. from a ruptured tubo-ovarian abscess.

Hare (1990b) suggests that the finding of chlamydia from the cervix is an acceptable alternative to the presumptive identification of gonococci.

The most important presenting symptom is abdominal pain. Weström and Mårdh (1990) suggest the pain is usually subacute in onset, bilateral, low abdominal or pelvic, and dull in character. However, Westcott (1992), when describing patients' stories, notes that many women have acute, severe pain when presenting to a doctor. It has been noted by various researchers that although pain is usually present in patients with PID, not all patients with pain have infection (MacLean, 1995). Detailed questions about the site and nature of the pain need to be asked, as pain from PID will often be present during menstruation, sexual intercourse and micturition. Some studies have found that women with PID have deep dyspareunia. However Stacey and Munday (1994) in their study found deep dyspareunia was more common in women without PID and women with PID were more likely to describe the pain as stabbing.

MacLean (1995) suggests that 35% of patients with PID will complain of irregular bleeding and Weström and Mårdh (1990) note that irregular bleeding was significantly more common with chlamydia-associated PID than with other causes of PID. They go on to suggest that with a young woman, a report of irregular uterine bleeding of recent onset should always suggest the presence of a genital infection (endometritis), especially if she is not taking an oral contraceptive. In one study about half of the patients with PID reported an increased or altered vaginal discharge, illustrating that the lower genital infection preceding PID may go unnoticed (Weström & Mårdh, 1990).

Patients who are acutely ill may also complain of nausea and vomiting, often associated with a high temperature. Some patients also have proctitis and pain on opening their bowels.

It has been noted that the diagnosis of PID becomes more accurate with the severity of the disease (Stacey & Munday, 1994). However, the clinical criteria used to diagnose PID vary greatly and Weström and Mårdh (1990) found that routine laparoscopy for the diagnosis of salpingitis revealed that commonly used criteria were correct in about 65% of cases only. Stacey and Munday (1994) studied 81 women attending a GUM clinic with mild to moderate, acute or chronic abdominal pain, to compare laparoscopically the clinical features of those who had PID with those who did not. They found PID in 14% laparoscopically, adhesions in 11% and endometriosis in 16%, and they concluded that women with PID were clinically indistinguishable from women with other diagnoses or no obvious cause. However, it should be noted that laparoscopic findings may be normal even when patients have objective evidence of endometritis and/or endosalpingitis (Weström & Mårdh, 1990).

In this country, most genito-urinary physicians and gynaecologists do not feel it is necessary to undertake laparoscopy routinely on women with a presumptive diagnosis of PID. MacLean (1995) suggests that laparoscopy is useful when there is unhelpful or equivocal microbiology and Hare (1990a) suggests that laparoscopy is highly desirable in the following cases:

1.   In a woman who is severely ill, especially if she is in cardiovascular shock.
2.   In a patient who is older, because the incidence of endometriosis or malignant disease is higher.
3.   When ectopic pregnancy is a possible diagnosis suggested by menstrual irregularity.

4.   In a woman who claims never to have had intercourse.
5.   If there is little or no response 72 hours after antibiotic treatment has started.

Many authors also suggest using laparoscopy to exclude a differential diagnosis such as ectopic pregnancy, appendicitis, bleeding from a corpus luteum or other pelvic conditions.

Treatment

Most authors suggest that women with severe infection or an unclear diagnosis should be treated in hospital. Weström and Mårdh (1990) suggest that if a woman is treated on an outpatient basis, as with most patients seen in GUM, the woman should rest at home, avoid sexual intercourse and monitor her temperature regularly. Obviously, where the patient is treated has an effect on the drug regimen used.

Hare (1990a) notes that in most cases of PID, antibiotic therapy will be started before a full microbiological picture is known and most people agree with this form of management. The choice of antibiotic is influenced by availability of the drug, local policy on prescribing and patient sensitivity, though most studies suggest triple or double regimens should be used to give a broad spectrum of antibacterial cover. The extent of presenting signs and symptoms will also affect antibiotic choice, as those patients who have acute peritonitis and systemic upset are more likely to have gonococcal, aerobic or anaerobic infection, while patients who present with milder symptoms are more likely to have chlamydia (MacLean, 1995).

MacLean (1995) uses the following descriptions of drugs used to treat PID.

Penicillins and cephalosporins

Penicillins and cephalosporins give good tissue penetration and various formulations of these drugs give good activity against gonococci, streptococci and many Gram-positive and Gram-negative aerobes and anaerobes.

Aminoglycosides

Aminoglycosides such as gentamycin and tobramycin are useful in severe infection but are ineffective against anaerobes or streptococci and they are also fairly toxic to the kidneys.

Tetracyclines

Tetracyclines give a wide spectrum of cover against most gonococci, Gram-negative aerobic organisms, chlamydia and most anaerobes. However they cannot be used during pregnancy.

Erythromycin

Erythromycin is effective against chlamydia and gonococci but less effective than the tetracyclines against other Gram-negative aerobes and anaerobes causing PID.

Metronidazole

Metronidazole is the most effective drug against serious anaerobic infection, though it has common side-effects of gastrointestinal upset and alcohol intolerance.

MacLean (1995) suggests the use of vibramycin if the patient is at home and erythromycin if the patient is pregnant. Hare (1990a) would use ampicillin or amoxycillin with probenecid plus doxycycline or something equivalent plus metronidazole, when treating outpatients. Weström and Mårdh (1990) recommend cefoxitin with probenecid or ceftriaxone or amoxycillin and probenecid followed by doxycycline, for women treated as outpatients. However, in the case of severe infection, they all agree that intravenous therapy must be started as an inpatient.

If the patient has an IUD it should be removed, except where there is the risk of pregnancy following intercourse within the preceding 48 hours when the woman is at or just after mid-cycle (Hare, 1990a).

Unless diagnostic laparoscopy is to be performed, surgery is likely to be needed to remove retained products of conception, to treat life-threatening disease, if conservative treatment has failed or if there is an abscess. Such surgery should include division of adhesions and peritoneal toilet and should be as conservative as possible without major excisions (Weström & Mårdh, 1990; MacLean, 1995).

Complications

Short-term complications of PID, such as abscess formation, have already been mentioned. Fitz-Hugh-Curtis syndrome comprises perihepatitis associated with PID, normally following gonococcal infection though some studies have shown an association with chlamydial infection. The patient with this syndrome will have tenderness of the upper right quadrant of the abdomen and diagnosis should be confirmed by laparoscopy, when oedema of the liver capsule and adhesions – referred to as 'piano-string' adhesions – between the capsule and the peritoneum may be seen (Hare, 1990a).

The long-term consequences of PID relate to post-infection damage to various structures in the pelvis. Chronic abdominal pain is a serious consequence of PID. The pain is described as dull, continuing, often cycle-related worsening around ovulation (Weström, 1988). In a study reported by Weström and Mårdh (1990), 18% of women who had been diagnosed with salpingitis and 5% of the controls reported abdominal pain lasting longer than 6 months causing them to seek medical help. Patients may also have dyspareunia, often severely, which can lead to relationship problems. Long term antibiotics do little to control pain and may encourage drug resistance. Painkillers may also be of limited use. Weström (1988) advises the use of drugs used to treat endometriosis, such as continuous danazol or progesterone therapy. However, many women will eventually ask for a surgical removal of uterus, tubes and ovaries, if they are involved, even though this means they cannot become pregnant (Weström, 1988; MacLean, 1995).

There have been many studies of infertility following PID, from which Weström (1988) notes various points. The younger a woman was when she first had PID, the more chance she has of getting pregnant later; the chance of becoming infertile following PID doubles with each new episode of PID; moderate or severe disease is more likely to lead to infertility than mild PID; PID associated with gonorrhoea causes less problems to fertility than non-gonococcal PID, though chlamydia was not known about until the later years of many of these studies. Before antibiotics were available, 50–75% of women were found to be infertile following PID. Therefore, if women are not treated nowadays, because their silent PID is not diagnosed, these rates of infertility may still occur. Moore and Cates (1990) note that there is an approximately 11% risk of infertility following one episode of PID, 23% risk following two episodes and over 50% risk following three episodes.

The risk of ectopic or tubal pregnancy following PID has also been well documented over the years. Various studies have shown an increase in the rate of ectopic pregnancies from the 1960s to present times. It must be remembered that the detection rate of ectopics has increased dramatically over that time, but it has also been shown that women who have had PID, have a seven- to 10-fold increased risk of ectopic pregnancy when compared to women who have never had

PID (Weström & Mårdh, 1990). Again there have been studies showing that women with ectopic pregnancies are more likely to have antibodies to chlamydia than women with intrauterine pregnancies.

Follow-up

The extreme importance of contact tracing of the sexual partners of women with PID cannot be overemphasised and all authors seem to agree on this point. Weström and Mårdh (1990) state that in all cases of PID the patient's sexual partner(s) should be examined, particularly for gonorrhoea and chlamydia, and treated if these pathogens are found. Kamwendo et al. (1993) found that gonorrhoea, chlamydia or NSU was demonstrated in 59.7% of the male partners of women with PID in their study. However, only 32% of the males with gonorrhoea or chlamydia and 8.5% of those with NSU had subjective symptoms of urethritis, which emphasises the need for clinical and laboratory examination of the sexual partners of women with PID.

Weström and Mårdh (1990), along with many other authors, have noted that there is strong evidence of an epidemic of 'silent' PID, but there is little information as yet on the size of the problem.

Rome (1994) points out that the high morbidity and high medical expenses resulting from the after-effects of PID mean that efforts at primary, secondary and tertiary prevention of PID are very important and should be intensified.

Conclusion

Strategies to control PID infection within the population must centre around controlling the spread of gonorrhoea and particularly chlamydia. Condom use should be encouraged. Women at risk of gonococcal or chlamydial infection should be screened before operative procedures such as termination of pregnancy that breach the cervical barrier, and partners of women with PID should be screened. This is the message GUM nurses should take forward.

Weström (1988) sums up by pointing out that a decreasing rate of serious long-term effects of PID can only be achieved by continuing research, education and day to day efforts to fight STDs.

Support group for women with PID

PID Support Network, c/o Women's Health Research and Information Centre, 52 Featherstone Street, London EC1Y 8RT. Tel: 0171 251 6580
Open Monday, Wednesday, Thursday and Friday, 10am–4pm.
Information leaflet, PID newsletter and telephone support network.

References

Berger RE, Alexander ER, Monda GD, Ansell J, McCormick G, Holmes KK (1978) *Chlamydia trachomatis* as a cause of acute 'idiopathic' epididymitis. New England Journal of Medicine 298(6): 301–4.

Brunham RC, Holmes KK, Embree JE (1990) Sexually transmitted diseases in pregnancy. In Holmes KK, Mårdh P-A, Sparling PF, Wiesner PJ (Eds), Sexually Transmitted Diseases, 2nd edn. New York: McGraw-Hill.

Cameron S (1993) A protocol for the detection of chlamydia. Nursing Standard 8(5): 25–7.

Crowley T, Milne D, Arumainayagam JT, Paul ID, Caul EO (1992) The laboratory diagnosis of male *Chlamydia trachomatis* infections – a time for change? Journal of Infection 25(supplement 1): 69–75.

Dawson CR, Schachter J, Ostler HB, Gilbert RM, Smith DE, Engleman EP (1970) Inclusion conjunctivitis and Reiter's syndrome in a married couple: chlamydial infections in a series of both diseases. Archives of Ophthalmology 83: 300–6.

DOH (1993) The Health of the Nation: Key Area Handbook HIV/AIDS and Sexual Health. London: HMSO.

DOH (1995) Sexually Transmitted Diseases, England 1994. Department of Health Statistical Bulletin. London: HMSO.

Dryden MS, Wilkinson M, Redman M, Millar MR (1994) Detection of *Chlamydia trachomatis* in general practice urine samples. British Journal of General Practice 44: 114–17.

Greendale GA, Haas ST, Holbrook K, Walsh B, Schachter J, Phillips RS (1993) The relationship of *Chlamydia trachomatis* infection and male infertility. American Journal of Public Health 83(7): 996–1001.

Hager WD, Eschenbach DA, Spence MR, Sweet RL (1983) Criteria for diagnosis and grading of salpingitis. Obstetrics and Gynecology 61(1): 113–14.

Hammerschlag MR, Handsfield HH, Judson FN (1987) When to suspect chlamydia. Patient Care (November 15): 64–78.

Hare J (1990a) Pelvic inflammatory disease. In Csonka GW, Oates JK (Eds), Sexually Transmitted Diseases – A Textbook of Genitourinary Medicine. London: Baillière Tindall.

Hare J (1990b) Pelvic inflammatory disease: current approaches and ideas. International Journal of STD & AIDS 1:393–400.

Harrison HR, Costin M, Meder JB, Bownds LM, Sim DA, Lewis M, Alexander ER (1985) Cervical *Chlamydia trachomatis* infection in university women: relationship to history, contraception, ectopy, and cervicitis. American Journal of Obstetrics and Gynecology 153(3): 244–51.

Hay PE, Thomas BJ, McKenzie P, Taylor-Robinson D (1993) Detection of *Chlamydia trachomatis* in men: sensitive tests for sensitive urethras. Sexually Transmitted Diseases 20(1): 1–4.

Kamwendo F, Johansson E, Moi H, Forslin L, Danielsson D (1993) Gonorrhoea, genital chlamydial infection, and nonspecific urethritis in male partners of women hospitalized and treated for acute pelvic inflammatory disease. Sexually Transmitted Diseases 20(3): 143–6.

Keat A, Rowe I (1990) Reiter's syndrome and reactive arthritis. In Csonka GW, Oates JK (Eds), Sexually Transmitted Diseases – A Textbook of Genitourinary Medicine. London: Baillière Tindall.

Keat A, Thomas B, Dixey J, Osborn M, Sonnex C, Taylor-Robinson D (1987) *Chlamydia trachomatis* and reactive arthritis: the missing link. The Lancet (January 10): 72–4

Kok T-W, Payne LE, Bailey SE, Waddell RG (1993) Urine and the laboratory diagnosis of *Chlamydia trachomatis* in males. Genitourinary Medicine 69: 51–3.

MacLean A (1995) Pelvic infection. In Whitfield C (Ed), Dewhurst's Textbook of Obstetrics and Gynaecology for Postgraduates, 5th edn. Oxford: Blackwell Science.

Mahony JB, Luinstra KE, Sellors JW, Chernesky MA (1990) Comparison of polymerase chain reaction (PCR), enzyme immunoassay and culture for the diagnosis of *C. trachomatis* infections in symptomatic and asymptomatic males and females. In Bowie RW, Caldwell HD, Jones RP, Mårdh P-A, Ridgway GL, Schachter J, Stamm WE, Ward ME (Eds), Chlamydia Infections. Cambridge: Cambridge University Press.

Moore D, Cates W (1990) Sexually transmitted diseases and infertility. In Holmes KK, Mårdh P-A, Sparling PF, Wiesner PJ (Eds), Sexually Transmitted Diseases, 2nd edn. New York: McGraw-Hill.

Nilsson S, Johannisson G, Lycke E (1981) Isolation of *Chlamydia trachomatis* from the urethra and from prostatic fluid in men with signs and symptoms of acute urethritis. In Johannisson G (1981) Studies of *C. trachomatis* as a Cause of Lower Urogenital Infection. Goteborg: Acta Dermato-venereologica (supplement 93).

Patel R, Kinghorn GR, Kudesia G, Van Hegan R (1991) *Chlamydia trachomatis* detection and non-invasive sampling methods. Lancet 338: 181.

Poletti F, Medici MC, Alinovi A, Menozzi MG, Sacchini P, Stagni G, Toni M, Benoldi D (1985) Isolation of *Chlamydia trachomatis* from the prostatic cells in patients affected by nonacute abacterial prostatitis. Journal of Urology 134: 691–3.

Ridgway GL, Taylor-Robinson D (1992) Current problems in microbiology: 1 Chlamydial infections: which laboratory test? Journal of Clinical Pathology 44: 1–5.

Rome ES (1994) Pelvic inflammatory disease in the adolescent. Current Opinion in Pediatrics 6: 383–7.

Schachter J (1990) Biology of *Chlamydia trachomatis*. In Holmes KK, Mårdh P-A, Sparling PF, Wiesner PJ (Eds), Sexually Transmitted Diseases, 2nd edn. New York: McGraw-Hill.

Stacey CM, Munday PE (1994) Abdominal pain in women attending a genitourinary medicine clinic: who has PID? International Journal of STD & AIDS 5: 338–42.

Stamm WE, Guinan ME, Johnson C, Starcher T, Holmes KK, McCormack WM (1984) Effect of treatment regimes for *Neisseria gonorrhoeae* on simultaneous infection with *Chlamydia trachomatis*. New England Journal of Medicine 310(9): 545–9.

Stamm WE, Holmes KK (1990) *Chlamydia trachomatis* infections of the adult. In Holmes KK, Mårdh P-A, Sparling PF, Wiesner PJ (Eds), Sexually Transmitted Diseases, 2nd edn. New York: McGraw-Hill.

Taylor-Robinson D (1992) The value of non-culture techniques for diagnosis of *Chlamydia trachomatis* infections: making the best of a bad job. European Journal of Microbiological Infectious Diseases 11(6): 499–503.

Westcott P (1992) Pelvic Inflammatory Disease and Chlamydia. London: Thorsons.

THE LIBRARY
KENT & SUSSEX HOSPITAL
TUNBRIDGE WELLS
KENT TN4 8AT

Weström L (1988) Long-term consequences of pelvic inflammatory disease. In Hare MJ (Ed), Genital Tract Infection in Women. Edinburgh: Churchill Livingstone.

Weström L, Mårdh P-A (1990) Acute pelvic inflammatory disease (PID). In Holmes KK, Mårdh P-A, Sparling PF, Wiesner PJ (Eds), Sexually Transmitted Diseases, 2nd edn. New York: McGraw-Hill.

Whelan M (1988) Nursing management of the patient with *Chlamydia trachomatis* infection. Nursing Clinics of North America 23(40): 877–83.

Wølner-Hanssen P, Kiviat NB, Holmes KK (1990) Atypical pelvic inflammatory disease: subacute, chronic, or subclinical upper genital tract infection in women. In Holmes KK, Mårdh P-A, Sparling PF, Wiesner PJ (Eds), Sexually Transmitted Diseases, 2nd edn. New York: McGraw-Hill.

Bibliography

Govan A, Hart D, Callander R (Eds) (1993) Gynaecology Illustrated, 4th edn. Edinburgh: Churchill Livingstone.

Saunders J (1988) Sexually transmitted diseases – chlamydia infection. Nursing Times 84(49): 35.

Sellors J, Mahony J, Jang D, Pickard L, Castriciano S, Landis S, Stewart I, Seidelman W, Cunningham I, Chernesky M (1991) Rapid, on-site diagnosis of chlamydial urethritis in men by detection of antigens in urethral swabs and urine. Journal of Clinical Microbiology 29(2): 407–9.

Stacey CM, Munday PE, Taylor-Robinson D, Thomas BJ, Gilchrist C, Ruck F (1992) A longitudinal study of pelvic inflammatory disease. British Journal of Obstetrics and Gynaecology 99: 994–9.

Taylor-Robinson D (1990) Clinical significance of genital chlamydia and mycoplasmal infections. In Csonka GW, Oates JK (Eds), Sexually Transmitted Diseases – A Textbook of Genitourinary Medicine. London: Baillière Tindall.

White K (1992) Sterile condition. Nursing Times 88(44): 34–6.

Chapter 7
Bacterial vaginosis, candidiasis and trichomoniasis

Mary Phillips, Christina McGlynn and Bernice Fagan

Introduction

Many women present in genito-urinary medicine (GUM) clinics complaining that they have noticed a greater amount of vaginal secretions or wetness at certain times of the month. It is important to point out to women that a discharge is quite normal and helps to keep the vagina clean.

The amount and consistency of the discharge varies at different times in the menstrual cycle (Peel & MacLean, 1995): the secretion is greatest at the midpoint between two periods, which is when ovulation can occur, and is at its least just before and just after menstruation.

Vaginal secretions also act as a lubricant during sexual intercourse, preventing friction and reducing soreness afterwards. This normal discharge usually presents as a clear or slightly cloudy secretion that feels slippery to the touch. When it dries it may be faintly yellow and cause slight staining on underwear. It is particularly noticeable mid-cycle, during pregnancy and in some women taking the oral contraceptive pill (Rein, 1990).

Three conditions that affect the vagina and vaginal discharge will now be discussed.

Bacterial vaginosis

Introduction

Bacterial vaginosis (BV) is one of the commonest reasons why women attend their general practitioner (GP) or GUM clinic. BV is an overgrowth of naturally occurring bacteria found in the vagina, which is characterised by a distinct lack of lactobacilli on microscopy and an increase in other bacteria that are usually only present in much smaller numbers. Eschenbach (1993) suggests that this syndrome is very important, because of its recently discovered relevance to upper genital tract infections.

Although Larsson, Platz-Christensen and Sundström (1991) found that women with BV have similar sexual behaviour to other women at risk of sexually transmitted diseases (STDs), Hill (1993) suggests that the pathogenesis of BV is still not fully investigated or understood.

Background and microbiology

The condition now known as BV has had an interesting history and has been known by various other names. In the last century, before technology to identify organisms present in vaginal flora was available, any vaginal infection that was not candida or trichomonas was termed non-specific vaginitis (Hill, 1993).

The presence of lactobacilli in normal vaginal flora was described at the end of the last century and it was understood that lactobacilli produce lactic acid, which keeps the vaginal pH low and therefore stops other organisms growing in the vagina (Eschenbach, 1993). Between 1914 and 1921, other bacteria were identified and found to be present in non-specific vaginitis.

Gardner and Dukes (1955) undertook work on vaginitis and identified a new organism, which they called *Haemophilus vaginalis*. They discovered that stippled squamous cells could be seen when the discharge of women with vaginitis was examined microscopically and they called this a clue to the diagnosis of *H. vaginalis* vaginitis, hence the use of the term 'clue cell'. They also described clinical features that are still used as a basis of diagnosis today, that is a raised pH, a grey homogenous discharge that smells and the lack of lactobacilli on microscopy. Eschenbach (1993) notes that although Gardner and Dukes isolated one organism that caused BV, they did not realise how complex the microbiology of BV actually is.

During the 1950s through to the 1970s a lot more work was done on BV. Hill (1993) states that the name was changed twice in this time, first to *Corynebacterium vaginale* and then to *Gardnerella vaginalis* – in recognition of the work done by Dr Gardner.

In the 1970s there were major breakthroughs in culturing anaerobic micro-organisms that allowed microbiologists to identify several anaerobic bacteria present with gardnerella (Eschenbach, 1993), and then further extensive work enabled researchers to differentiate the organisms present.

Dawson (1990) notes that the organisms usually associated with BV are *Gardnerella vaginalis* and *Mycoplasma hominis*, which are facultative anaerobes, and anaerobes such as *Bacteroides* species, peptostreptococci and peptococci. *Mobiluncus* species have also been found, but their relevance is not known (Dawson, 1990). Hill (1993) notes that *Ureaplasma urealyticum* has also been found in non-specific vaginitis.

The presence of so many aerobic and anaerobic bacteria led to the decision to change the name of the condition again, to bacterial vaginosis, as the term vaginosis is usual when bacteria are associated with the cause of a vaginal infection. Eschenbach (1993) notes that vaginitis is inflammation of the vaginal epithelium, with many leukocytes being produced, and because BV is a bacterial infection, it does not cause inflammation of the vaginal epithelium. Also, the term BV suggests that a smell or odour is present, and this is a common complaint of patients with this condition (Eschenbach, 1993).

Complications

Hill (1993) notes that although BV itself is generally not considered serious, recent research has shown involvement of BV with upper genital tract infections and conditions such as post-partum endometritis and premature rupture of the membranes (PROM) (Dawson, 1990; Eschenbach, 1993). It has also been shown that BV organisms such as *Gardnerella vaginalis* and *Mycoplasma hominis* are found in clinical chorioamnionitis or amniotic fluid infection (Gibbs, 1993).

Other research has shown that BV may be particularly associated not only with PROM, but also with premature labour and birth and that factors such as proteases, which help the transport of bacteria to foetal membranes and therefore damage them, may be produced by BV organisms (McGregor, French & Seo 1993). Gibbs (1993) notes that trials are being carried out to see if treating BV reduces such complications in pregnancy.

Clinical features

BV is one of the few infections that is diagnosed mainly through clinical features. The main features of BV are an increase in vaginal discharge, which is usually grey or white, homogeneous or uniform in character and has a fishy malodorous smell (Dawson, 1990).

However, there is rarely any inflammation or vaginitis, so there is little discomfort with BV. Some women notice an increase in malodour around the time of menstruation or after sexual intercourse, which can be explained by the release of amines caused by semen and blood working in a similar way to potassium hydroxide when added to vaginal discharge (Bowman, 1993).

Easmon, Hay and Ison (1992) suggest that about 50% of women attending GUM clinics who have BV are asymptomatic and that BV is more common than either candidiasis or *Trichomonas vaginalis* (TV) infection in women who attend because of an abnormal discharge.

Tests for BV

There is no laboratory culture test available at present to diagnose this condition. Although there has been extensive research undertaken to distinguish and identify the organisms present in BV, there has been no change in the way it is diagnosed. The diagnosis is made by finding three out of the four criteria proposed by Amsel et al. (1983), and which are listed below:

1.   homogeneous, grey/white discharge;
2.   characteristic fishy smell when potassium hydroxide (KOH) 10% is added to the vaginal discharge – usually referred to as the sniff, whiff or amine test;
3.   vaginal discharge with a pH of 4.5 and above;
4.   clue cells present on microscopy.

Vaginal discharge

The physical examination prior to insertion of the speculum may be an important indicator, as this may show a moist, white/grey discharge covering the labia minora and sometimes the labia majora and introitus (Dawson, 1990). When the speculum is introduced, there may be a homogenous, thin, white/grey discharge coating the vaginal walls, which may be so thinly coated that it only shows as a change in light reflex, or there may be a discharge heavy enough to cause pooling in the posterior fornix and bubbles may be seen in the discharge (Rein, 1990). Easmon, Hay and Ison (1992) suggest that the lack of an abnormal discharge does not exclude a diagnosis of BV. A fishy smell may be noted, though there is rarely any erythema or inflammation unless there is a concomitant infection (Rein, 1990).

The sniff, whiff or amine test

This involves the mixing of vaginal discharge with the alkali 10% KOH, either on a glass slide (Dawson, 1990) or straight on to the speculum. If it is to be mixed on a slide, the wet preparation (prep) sample may be used after looking for TV, though it is easier to take a separate sample specifically for this.

At whatever stage this test is performed, a few drops of KOH are added and the sample sniffed immediately, as a positive result is indicated by a transient, quickly released fishy odour (Dawson, 1990). The fishy odour is explained by Brand and Galask (1986) as being due to the release of volatile polyamines from their salts by the addition of alkali and in particular the release of trimethylamine, which is the predominant contributor to the smell of rotting fish.

It is possible to obtain a false positive amine test if the woman has recently had sexual intercourse, not only because the volatile amine putrescine is found in semen, but also because semen has a high pH and releases amines; some women are so sensitive to the smell that they can smell it without having BV (Easmon, Hay & Ison 1992). Douching, recent bathing or recent removal of a vaginal tampon may also give a false positive KOH result.

Vaginal pH

Dawson (1990) states that the normal pH of the vagina is 4.2 or less and a pH of 4.5 or above is taken as being diagnostic of BV. Different techniques can be used for measuring the pH of the vaginal discharge, such as pH paper or indicator strips.

There are various ways of placing a sample of discharge on the pH paper or strip. One method is to clip a piece of paper, approximately 3 centimetres long, to a pair of forceps and to dip this into the discharge present in the posterior fornix or the discharge present on the speculum when it has been removed. Many people take a sample of discharge with a loop and either put it on a glass slide and dip the paper or indicator strip into it or just apply the loop sample directly to the paper (Dawson, 1990) or indicator strip.

If water is used to warm the speculum or water-based gel is used to lubricate it, the pH can be altered and it is important to test the vaginal discharge, not the water. Blood will alter the pH of the vagina, so it is important to note the presence of blood when testing the pH (Dawson, 1990). Both blood and water will give a pH above 4.5.

Easmon, Hay and Ison (1992) describe finding a pH of more than 4.5 as a sensitive indicator of BV infection, though TV can also cause the pH to be raised (Rein, 1990). Care must be taken not to measure cervical secretions (Dawson, 1990), as these always have a pH of more than 6.0.

Clue cells

As the pH increases, the anaerobic bacteria present in BV stick to the vaginal epithelial cells more strongly (Easmon, Hay & Ison 1992). When the sample taken from the vagina is Gram-stained and viewed under the microscope, the epithelial cells will appear to be granulated (Gardner & Dukes, 1955). Clue cells may be so coated with cocco-bacillary bacteria that the borders become obscured and even the nucleus may be obscured.

A wet mount slide can also be examined for clue cells, though the use of both wet and Gram-stained slides is more reliable (Dawson, 1990). Finding and recognising clue cells on a slide is one of the most specific criteria for diagnosing BV, though it is dependent on the microscopist's skill in recognising clue cells (Easmon, Hay & Ison 1992). The way a slide is stained, whether it is heated too much and the presence of debris or degenerate cells may all affect clue cell recognition. Figure 7.1 shows a diagram of a clue cell and a normal epithelial cell.

Easmon, Hay and Ison (1992) note that 81% of women attending a GUM clinic with BV had clue cells, as did 6% of women who did not have BV. An asymptomatic woman who has clue cells but none of the other criteria for BV should not be treated for BV (Rein, 1990). It has been suggested by Eschenbach et al. (1988) that for the test to be positive, 20% or more of the epithelial cells should have the appearance of clue cells.

There is a marked absence of lactobacilli on a slide when BV is present and no pus cells are seen (Dawson, 1990), unless there is a co-existing infection present. It is very important to look closely for gonorrhoea if pus cells are seen.

Treatment

Metronidazole orally and clindamycin cream vaginally are the two standard treatments for BV nowadays, though other treatments have been and are still sometimes used.

Metronidazole 400 mg twice a day for 5–7 days is used to treat BV, though sometimes a stat dose of 2 g can be given instead of a week-long course (Dawson, 1990). Metronidazole is an antimicrobial drug with selective activity against anaerobic bacteria by interfering with the activity of their DNA (Hopkins, 1992).

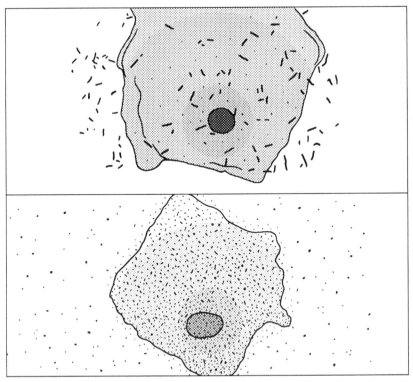

Figure 7.1: Normal epithial cell with lactobacilli (above): a clue cell (below).

However, metronidazole can have side effects. These include darkening of the urine, especially with the 2 g stat dose; nausea; a metallic taste in the mouth; and drowsiness and dizziness (Turner & Richens, 1978; Hopkins, 1992). In addition, patients can be profoundly sick if they drink alcohol while on metronidazole and it is advisable to warn them not to drink alcohol for up to 24 hours after finishing the course (Dawson, 1990). Turner and Richens (1978) note that metronidazole acts like disulfiram (antabuse), which is used in the treatment of alcoholism and which acts by blocking the metabolism of alcohol at the acetaldehyde formation stage. Therefore, it is important that nurses explain the side effects when giving metronidazole to patients.

Godley (1993) states that metronidazole should not be given during the first trimester of pregnancy, though Hopkins (1992) notes that it has been given during pregnancy. Lossick (1990) suggests that lactobacilli are allowed to regrow when metronidazole is given, which is essential for restoring the normal balance of vaginal flora and Rein (1990) states that metronidazole has been reported as curing over 90% of BV.

Clindamycin cream 2% is generally prescribed for daily treatment for 7 days; it is supplied in a 40 g tube with seven disposable applicators. The cream is squeezed into an applicator until the plunger reaches the stopping point and it is then inserted into the vagina at night for 7 nights, using a new applicator each night. However, a recent pilot study by Dhar et al. (1994) has shown that 2% clindamycin cream for just 3 days is a safe and effective treatment for BV. Ahmed-Jushuf, Shahmanesh and Arya (1995) conducted a larger multicentre trial, which backed up the findings of Dhar et al. and found that 2% clindamycin cream was well tolerated and effective in treating BV. The treatment should not be given to women who are sensitive to clindamycin, linomycin or any of the components of the vaginal cream, one of which is mineral oil, which may also weaken latex and rubber products such as condoms and diaphragms. The product information recommends that condoms and diaphragms should not be used within 72 hours of treatment and also, that if women have diarrhoea while using clindamycin cream, they should stop the treatment immediately, because about 5% of the dose is absorbed systemically from the vagina (Upjohn, 1992).

Other treatments that may be given for BV include the use of chlorhexidine pessaries, which was investigated by Ison et al. (1987), who found that this treatment was as effective as metronidazole in curing BV. Nayagam et al. (1992) found that ofloxacin 200 mg twice daily for 7 days was a safe and effective alternative to metronidazole. However, Boeke et al. (1993) found that lactic acid suppositories did not treat BV, though many patients appeared to recover without any active treatment at all.

Follow-up and patient education

Recurrent BV can be very upsetting (Easmon, Hay & Ison 1992) and it is important that women with repeated infections have swabs taken to establish a diagnosis, so that the correct treatment can be given. Aggravating factors such as douching, which disturbs the natural flora; tight clothing; strong detergents, bath oils and bubble baths; strong soaps; and vaginal deodorants should be eliminated, and women may need to stop using tampons.

There has been a lot of research looking at the male partners of women with BV. Dawson (1990) suggests that caution should be used in treating male partners, as BV cannot be proved to be an STD and it is important not to suggest infidelity. However, Adler (1990) states that male contacts should be seen, as BV may be sexually acquired, especially if the woman has recurrent attacks. Moi et al. (1989) found that treating the sexual contacts of women with BV did not improve the cure rate in women with recurrent BV.

Bowman (1993) believes that as semen leads to a release of amines, using a condom during episodes of BV may reduce the exacerbation of odour and discharge. However, she does not believe that sexual transmission is the biggest cause of recurrence, though it may introduce the organisms initially, but that changes in the vaginal flora are important.

Cook et al. (1992) found residual abnormalities in the biochemistry and vaginal flora in women following treatment of BV and they believe that this supports the idea that recurrence of BV, particularly in the early stages, is a relapse rather than a new infection and that possibly further treatment should be given to such women.

It is also important to consider the implications for women with BV who have sex with other women. Research into this has been undertaken at two clinics in London which run sexual health services for lesbians. These clinics were set up in 1992 and 1993 to deal with previously unaddressed sexual health needs of lesbians and to offer information about sexual transmission of infections between lesbians. BV is much more likely to be passed between two women than between a woman and a man, as their biological make-up is the same. Conway and Humphries (1994) note that 47% of the women seen at their clinic for lesbian women were found to have BV, though there were many factors involved in the aetiology, and the role of sexual transmission was unclear.

When taking a sexual history, it is important to establish the sex of the partner very early on in the consultation. The doctor needs to avoid questions such as 'Do you have a boyfriend?', as this may lead to the patient feeling uncomfortable about revealing their sexuality. The doctor or interviewer needs to be aware of issues relevant to lesbians and if they are not, they should seek advice or refer the patient to a colleague who is aware. Nurses should be sensitive to the needs of lesbians and provide them with a safe environment (Conway & Humphries, 1994). It may be advisable to consider treating the woman's partner(s), as there may be a greater possibility of passing BV from woman to woman through lesbian sex.

It is useful to reiterate to all women with BV that it arises from an imbalance of bacteria that are usually present in the normal vaginal flora. Also, that although it may be sexually transmitted, that is not the most common way for it to occur, and it can occur in women who are not currently sexually active.

How much a patient understands about BV will depend on the approach of the doctor, nurse or other health care professional responsible for explaining the condition to them. Some women view BV as an STD and if they constantly come back with recurrences, it is very important they are given a full explanation.

If a woman has repeated recurrences of BV as part of her menstrual cycle, prophylactic treatment of 2 g single doses of metronidazole may be given (Bowman, 1993) after excluding all other reasons for recurrences. It is always important to establish that treatment has been complied with and that the patient has understood what BV is and all the factors that can affect the normal balance of vaginal flora. Much of the compliance and understanding by the patient is reliant on the information given in the GUM clinic, therefore it is very important that nurses are fully aware of what BV is and its implications.

Candidiasis

Background information

Candidiasis, also called candidosis, is commonly known as thrush. It is usually caused by a yeast fungus called *Candida albicans*, which can be found in the mouth, digestive tract and vagina and which is found in over 70% of cases of genital candidiasis (Csonka, 1990a). Woolley (1995a) believes that only a few women develop symptomatic infection, though up to 75% carry yeasts.

Kennedy (1995) notes that there are two forms of thrush: spores, which cause asymptomatic colonisation and spread; and mycelia or hyphae, which are produced when germination occurs. It appears that symptomatic vulvovaginitis, following invasion of tissue, is related to the germination stage of thrush (Kennedy, 1995), though both forms are often found together and the hyphal form seems to be more resistant to treatment and better at penetrating host tissue (Woolley, 1995b).

Candida in men causes balanitis or balano-posthitis (Dockerty & Sonnex, 1995). Both men and women may have asymptomatic thrush, with many different factors leading to recurrences in both sexes (Csonka,1990a).

Candida is not generally considered to be an STD, though sexual intercourse may lead to trauma causing damage to the vulva, which allows candida to penetrate the deeper layers of the vulval mucosa (Woolley, 1994). It is thought that 75% of women will have at least one episode of vaginal thrush at some time in their lives (Brockhurst & Mindel, 1993) and Csonka (1990a) divides women into two groups – those with recurrent, chronic candidiasis and those who have one or a few attacks. Kennedy (1995) also suggests that some women never have symptomatic thrush, even though they have candida present in their vaginas and therefore it appears that some kind of host defect may have a bearing on the occurrence of symptomatic thrush.

Precipitating factors

Candida thrives in warm, moist conditions, such as those found in the vagina (Woolley, 1995a). It is suggested that wearing nylon underwear, which is non-porous, can precipitate thrush (Peel & MacLean, 1995) by trapping body heat and perspiration and preventing air from circulating around the genital area. Poor hygiene, from not drying properly after washing and heavy sweating, may also lead to repeated attacks of thrush.

Kennedy (1995) states that there is anecdotal evidence that douching or using perfumes or scented soaps may contribute to candidiasis by altering the vaginal flora. Rashid, Collins and Kennedy (1991) considered the role of fomites or objects which transfer infection, such as underwear, and decided that they were not significant in causing recurrent thrush.

Pregnancy seems to predispose women to develop thrush, particularly in the third trimester, and it is thought that the increased level of glycogen in the cells of the vaginal epithelium and reduced cell-mediated immunity both have a role (Csonka, 1990a). High oestrogen contraceptive pills are also thought to lead to thrush (Kennedy, 1995), though other researchers including Rashid, Collins and Kennedy (1991) have found that modern oral contraceptives do not cause candidiasis, particularly those with a low dose of oestrogen (Woolley, 1994).

It has been known for many years that antibiotic treatment is linked to the development of thrush in some women. Antibiotics such as cephalosporins, penicillin and tetracyclines reduce the level of lactobacilli in the vagina (Csonka, 1990a), which allows candida to germinate more freely and take over the vaginal flora (Kennedy, 1995).

Diabetes mellitus in women is believed to be a factor contributing to recurrent attacks of thrush and this is thought to be due to increased numbers of large epithelial cells and raised levels of vaginal glycogen (Kennedy, 1995). However, although women with diabetes may have more asymptomatic candida, unless the diabetes is badly controlled, they do not appear to have more symptomatic infection (Woolley, 1994). It is also believed that abnormal levels of serum iron may have an effect in candidiasis (Kennedy, 1995).

Some observers think that the fact that the vagina is close to the anus may have an influence on genital candidiasis, however Rashid, Collins and Kennedy (1991) felt that yeasts in the mouth or rectum had no effect on the recurrence or clearance of vulvovaginal candidiasis. Finally, people who are immunocompromised, either from the effects of drugs, cancer or HIV infection, are often prone to recurrent outbreaks of candidiasis (Woolley, 1994).

It has been shown that candida can be found by culture from the vagina in about 20% of asymptomatic women, acting as a commensal, and it appears that candida will only produce a symptomatic infection in these women when the normal vaginal flora is disturbed, such as with antibiotics (Brockhurst & Mindel, 1993).

Men have much less candida infection than women generally. Balanitis resulting from candida is much less common than candidal vulvovaginitis, though candida infection may be recurrent in some men. Particular predisposing factors include a lack of penile hygiene, a tight foreskin and diabetes (Brockhurst & Mindel, 1993). Balanitis associated with candida is often due to an allergic response to yeasts present in the vaginal discharge of the man's sexual partner (Robertson, McMillan & Young, 1989). Uncircumcised men are more likely than circumcised men to acquire a candida infection, though they may be asymptomatic. Csonka (1990a) notes that candidal infection may be passed between practising male homosexuals with penile or anal infection.

Clinical features in women

One of the most common features of thrush in symptomatic women is vulvovaginal pruritus, which may vary from being slight to intolerable (Robertson, McMillan & Young, 1989). This vulval itch, combined with soreness, often occurs with an increased vaginal discharge. Thrush discharge may be thick, white and look like cottage cheese; this curdy looking discharge may be found in 70% of pregnant women and in 20% of non-pregnant women with thrush (Robertson, McMillan & Young, 1989). However, the discharge may be slight or absent and is very variable, from a homogenous thickness to a more watery discharge (Kennedy, 1995).

Examination of the genitalia often reveals oedema of the labia minora; this is common in thrush seen in pregnancy and sometimes fissures can be seen at the fourchette and anus (Robertson, McMillan & Young, 1989). Csonka (1990a) notes that patients may become excoriated from scratching at the itch. Erythema is a common sign of candida and is usually found on the mucocutaneous surfaces between the labia minora, though sometimes it can be seen on the labia majora, perineum and perianal skin (Robertson, McMillan & Young, 1989).

Rein (1990) notes that papules or papulopustules may be seen just beyond the main erythematous area. Up to 20% of women may also have a very red vagina and there may be superficial ulceration with bleeding present underneath, if plaques or patches of thrush are removed from the vagina. Some patients may complain of dryness, while others complain of a burning sensation, especially on micturition. This is more likely to occur if there is local excoriation due to scratching, though it may be wrongly attributed to cystitis (Robertson, McMillan & Young, 1989).

Kennedy (1995) notes that superficial dyspareunia may be present, causing worry and distress to the patient, and that occasionally there is so much vulvitis that it is impossible to use a speculum to examine the patient.

Clinical features in men

As previously mentioned, candida in men is far less common than in women, though in some men it can be recurrent. Dockerty and Sonnex (1995) note that penile irritation, with mild erythema and papules that are small and irregular, are common. Soreness and itching of the penis may be accompanied by a discharge from under the prepuce.

Robertson, McMillan and Young (1989) suggest that balanitis or balano-posthitis with superficial erosions may be found on examination and occasionally eroded maculopapular lesions and preputial oedema can be present. Men often complain of a burning sensation, particularly after sexual intercourse, and present with a transient rash (Kennedy, 1995).

Csonka (1990a) notes that if balano-posthitis is left untreated, the infection may spread to the scrotal area and produce a glazed-skin appearance.

Diagnosis and tests

It is essential to check the urine for sugar, as candidiasis is a not infrequent presentation of diabetes, and a random blood sugar test can also be useful. To make a diagnosis of vulvovaginal or penile candidiasis, a full history of the patient's condition is taken and documented and this is followed by an examination of the genital area with the appropriate specimens being taken (Kennedy, 1995), including slides for microscopy and culture plates with the appropriate medium.

Various culture media are used, one of which is Sabouraud's glucose agar. This is highly acid with a pH of 5.5 which inhibits the growth of bacteria (Robertson, McMillan & Young, 1989). Adler (1990) notes that Stuart's or Amies's media may be used to transport specimens, if necessary, and that further tests may need to be carried out to determine the exact species of candida.

Peel and MacLean (1995) feel that it is better to take a skin scraping from the vulva than a swab from the skin or that tape can be used to strip off cells, which are then put on a glass slide. Dockerty and Sonnex (1995) investigated the use of double-sided tape, applied to a slide, to take a specimen from the glans and sub-prepuce and found this method increased the sensitivity of microscopy in diagnosing candida in men.

In women it is essential to use a speculum inserted into the vagina when obtaining a specimen for microscopy, as this enables the doctor or nurse to thoroughly examine and view the vagina and any discharge. A plastic loop is used to take a sample from the posterior fornix or from a plaque in the vagina for a dry and a wet preparation as described in Chapter 1.

The dry slide is Gramstained as described in Chapter 1 and it is important to note that all yeasts stain Gram-positive. Candida can be seen as Gram-positive blastophores or oval budding cells and as hyphae (Csonka, 1990a) under high-power oil immersion magnification.

The wet preparation can be examined with low-power magnification and TV infection can be excluded by this method as well. Adding the specimen to 5–10% potassium hydroxide, rather than saline, allows candida to be seen more clearly and reveals oval spores and hyphae (Kennedy, 1995).

Treatment

Kennedy (1995) notes that since the 1950s, topical antifungal therapy has commonly been prescribed for up to 2 weeks for the treatment of vaginal candidiasis. However, it is well known that many women do not comply with such treatment. Table 7.1 shows the topical and systemic drugs used to treat candidiasis.

Table 7.1: Vaginal and oral treatment for candidiasis

Drug	Route	Dosage	Side effects	Contraindications
Clotrimazole	Intravaginally	500 mg pessary – single dose 600 mg course – 6 x 100 mg pessaries, nightly for six consecutive nights 1 x 200 mg pessary on three consecutive nights	Occasional local irritation	None noted - the effect on latex condoms and diaphragms not yet known
Clotrimazole vaginal cream 2% (with a 5 g applicator)	Intravaginally	5 g x twice daily for three nights or 1 x 5 g nightly for six nights	As above	As above
Clotrimazole vaginal cream 10% (applicator as above)	Intravaginally	Single dose and may be used at night	As above	As above
Econazole cream (Ecostatin)	Intravaginally	150 mg per night for three nights or 150 mg as a stat dose	Occasional local irritation	Known to damage latex condoms and diaphragms
Miconazole	Intravaginally	1.2 g pessary – single dose at night	As above	As above
Miconazole cream 2%	Topically	Apply twice daily	As above	As above
Nystatin	Intravaginally	100 000 unit pessaries (1–2) inserted at night for 14–28 nights	As above	As above
Fluconazole (Diflucan)	Orally	150 mg stat	Usually related to gastrointestinal tract upsets, may cause nausea, abdominal pain	Should be used with caution in patients known to have hepatic disease NOT to be given in pregnancy
Itraconazole (Sporanex)	Orally	100 mg x 2 coated capsules twice daily for one day	May cause gastro-intestinal disturbances reported as mild	As above

Many different topical creams and pessaries are available. These are either polyenes such as nystatin or imidazoles, which include clotrimazole, econazole and others (Rein, 1990). Patient compliance is extremely important and Woolley (1994) notes that as clotrimazole is now available without prescription, many women treat themselves and attend their GP if the topical treatment does not work, leading to the use of oral therapy instead. However, oral therapy is now available without prescription as well.

Nystatin is a well established treatment. It has the side effect of staining clothing yellow (Robertson, McMillan & Young, 1989), and the long regimen of 2 weeks' treatment has led to lack of compliance by patients, with the result that imidazoles in shorter courses are normally prescribed now (Rein, 1990).

Adler (1990) notes that the imidazole drugs (clotrimazole, econazole and miconazole) are effective in shorter courses, often 3 days or even as single doses, which improves patient compliance. Topical cream may be used at the same time if there is vulval irritation.

There are now various oral treatments for thrush, which tend to improve patient compliance (Kennedy, 1995). Tobin, Leo and Granger (1992) found that treatment with itraconozole capsules, 200 mg twice in 24 hours, was as effective as a single dose treatment with 500 mg of clotrimazole in treating vaginal candida. Woolley (1994) notes that non-albicans *Candida* species, normally *Candida glabrota*, causes 5–16% of vaginal candidiasis and itraconazole has been found to be more potent against these than fluconazole.

It is important that patients on oral antifungal drugs are aware of possible side effects, so that they can inform their doctor if any problems arise during treatment. Patients on long-term oral therapy should be closely monitored (Sobel, 1986). However, it should be noted that patients who experience side effects on long-term therapy are often patients with HIV/AIDS and these patients are strictly monitored by their doctors.

Treatment in pregnancy

Pregnant women with candidiasis can be treated with local therapy, the same as non-pregnant women, but oral preparations are contraindicated (Godley, 1993). Candida has very little effect on a pregnancy with only occasional reports of candidal chorio-amniotitis. In the baby, intrapartum transmission can cause candidosis and skin infections such as nappy rash.

Follow-up tests

Normal follow-up tests for patients who have had a positive micro-scopic and culture diagnosis for candida may consist of any of the following:

1.   post treatment – if no further clinical features, signs and symp-toms are present, no further tests are needed unless the patient requests follow-up tests, in which case a wet/dry slide may be repeated to ensure there is no longer candidal infection present on microscopy;
2.   if the patient still has symptoms of a discharge – repeat only the wet/dry slides and culture for candida, unless the patient has had sexual intercourse with a new partner, in which case a full screen should be carried out to eliminate other infections as the cause of the symptomatic discharge.

Recurrent candidiasis

Woolley (1995b) suggests that at least four mycologically proven symptomatic episodes in the previous 12 months is considered a reasonable definition of recurrent vulvovaginal candidiasis, though Peel and MacLean (1995) suggest three episodes in a 12-month period.

Although some researchers believe that vaginal infection may occur as a result of a source of infection in the gut, Rein (1990) believes that support for re-infection from the rectum is lacking. Rashid, Collins and Kennedy (1991) considered the role of oral sex in transmission and found that there was no evidence that oral sex influenced treatment failure or had a definite role in recurrent infec-tion, even though 37% of women in their study had oral thrush and 65% of the patients said they regularly practised cunnilingus and/or fellatio. Woolley (1995b) states that there is still no absolute proof that sexual transmission causes recurrent infection.

Recurrence of thrush in women tends to begin during the week before menstruation and there may be no prior warning before severe vulval and vaginal pruritus and sometimes a discharge occur (Woolley, 1995b). These symptoms can be very distressing to the patients, as they often affect their sleeping pattern, adding to the emotional stress, which in turn can be a factor in recurrent candidal infections.

Chronic infection may cause lichenification, or thickening of the skin, around the vulval area (Woolley, 1995b); this is usually caused by intensive scratching, and treating the underlying precipitating factor allows the vulval area to return to normal. The budding yeast cells and hyphae forms of candida have both been found in infected tissue and Schnell (1982) found that hyphae can not only enter squamous epithelial cells in large numbers, but also to some depth, 15 cell layers down in the vaginal wall. Csonka (1990a) notes that these findings may account for the recurrences of vaginal candida, as the organism can remain deep in the vaginal tissue protected from topical antifungal treatment, then re-emerge into the vagina some weeks or months later when the epithelial cells are shed.

Women who have recurrent infection often have symptoms but minimal signs on examination, which is not really understood. It has been suggested that an allergic reaction may be involved, as occasionally the partner of a woman with candida will have irritation and soreness very soon after intercourse (Woolley, 1995b).

Csonka (1990a) discusses the role of a defective or suppressed T-lymphocyte response to candida, which may cause suppresser lymphocytes specific to candida to block the immune response, though the exact role of T-cell-mediated response is not clear (Woolley, 1995b).

Geiger, Foxman and Sobel (1995) believe that cultures are important in preventing misdiagnosis of recurrent thrush and in detecting yeasts which are not *Candida albicans*.

Management of recurrent thrush

Some women with recurrent thrush have problems relating to depression and psychosexual difficulties, and often dyspareunia following an acute episode of infection leads to fear that intercourse will be painful, which can then reduce normal vaginal lubrication (Woolley, 1995b). Treatment and eradication of underlying factors such as diabetes or long term antibiotics for acne is very important.

Information that women should be given to try and prevent recurrent attacks of candida includes:

1.   avoid wearing tights, underwear not made of cotton, leggings, lycra shorts and tight jeans or trousers;
2.   use sanitary towels rather than tampons when menstruating;
3.   avoid perfumed soaps, genital sprays, deodorants and any other irritants, such as bubble bath and disinfectants;
4.   wash and wipe the genital area from front to back;

5.   if an antibiotic must be taken, ask for treatment for thrush at the same time;

6.   make sure that the vagina is well lubricated during intercourse to reduce trauma.

General hygiene factors such as drying the vulva properly after bathing or swimming, ensuring the vulva is washed every day, wearing clean underwear and avoiding scratching are also important. The use of oral contraceptive drugs high in oestrogen should be avoided, though the role of modern low oestrogen dose pills is uncertain (Woolley, 1995b).

As previously mentioned, thrush may be passed on during sexual intercourse and the partners of women who have recurrent thrush should be checked for thrush, as they may be asymptomatic (Csonka, 1990a). However, Brockhurst and Mindel (1993) note that treating asymptomatic partners does not reduce infection or carriage in women.

It is important to acknowledge that resistant vaginal infection does not seem to be the sole factor in chronic and recurrent vulvovaginal candidiasis. Other factors that may be responsible for precipitating the infection should be eliminated before prescribing repeat prescriptions for short courses of treatment that may allow the patient to start treatment at the onset of an attack of thrush (Woolley, 1995b). He notes that self-initiated treatment will be better complied with if it is oral therapy and if the woman can make an accurate diagnosis of her two or three attacks a year.

Some women may benefit from counselling, to enable them to come to terms with the fact that long-term treatment may be required to prevent recurrence of candida infection. This will also give the patient the opportunity to discuss any psychosexual problems she may be experiencing, relating to the regular recurrence of thrush and how it affects her life. Long-term support may be needed with advice and reassurance that nearly all cases will be controlled.

Various prophylaxis regimens for recurrent candida have been suggested. Sanz and Hernanz (1987) suggested itraconazole 200 mg daily for 1–3 days. Fong (1992) found that treatment with clotrimazole was more effective than itraconazole when given daily for 5 days, then twice weekly for 6 months. Also, Fong, Bannatyne and Wong (1993) note that recurrent vaginal candidiasis is not linked to development of resistance to imidazoles.

Finally, it is important to recognise that despite candida not being classified as an STD, it is often one of the commonest complaints that women present with in GUM clinics and is frequently the cause of extreme distress to many women who attend for treatment and advice. Nurses caring for such patients should be supportive, sympathetic and offer general health education and advice on how to carry out self-help and preventive measures, in order to prevent recurrences of candida, while reiterating that there is much to be gained by seeking prompt medical advice and treatment if symptoms persist and current treatment is not helping.

Trichomoniasis

Background and aetiology

Although there has been a marked decrease in the incidence of trichomoniasis, it remains a very prevalent non-viral STD worldwide. Csonka (1990b) notes that the World Health Organization believes that there are about 180 million cases annually worldwide. Trichomoniasis is caused by the protozoan *Trichomonas vaginalis* (TV), which affects both sexes and can be isolated from the vagina, urethra and bladder in women and the urethra, glans penis, prostate and seminal vesicles in men, though urogenital infection in men rarely occurs outside the urethra (Rein & Müller, 1990).

TV is a single-celled organism that has four anterior flagellae and one posterior flagellum, which is embedded in an undulating membrane (Heine & McGregor, 1993), and these flagellae give the organism its mobility with characteristic jerky movements. Csonka (1990b) also notes that the protozoan has a large nucleus and a posterior axostyle which sticks out as a spine. TV varies in size from about the size of a pus cell to that of an epithelial cell and is generally ovoid, though it may be round or pyriform depending on where it is (Csonka, 1990b).

Prevalence and epidemiology

Csonka (1990b) notes that although TV can survive for short periods of time outside the body in moist areas, it is virtually always sexually transmitted and may coexist with other STDs. Women with trichomoniasis are likely to have another STD, such as chlamydia, gonorrhoea or BV (Wølner-Hanssen et al., 1989) and it is important to screen for other STDs.

The amount of sexual activity affects the prevalence of TV. Rein and Müller (1990) found that 50–70% of prostitutes, 13–25% of gynaecology clinic patients and 5% of women attending family planning clinics had TV infection. There is a fairly high incidence in the 30–40 year age group, as well as a peak incidence in 20–30 year olds (Csonka, 1990b). The incubation period is usually between 3 and 21 days and Csonka (1990b) has observed that it is commonly 7 days.

Clinical features in women

Many patients with TV are asymptomatic and Csonka (1990b) notes that 10–50% of women are thought to be either asymptomatic or to have such mild symptoms that TV infection is not suspected. In pregnancy, the number of asymptomatic infections may be even higher and Heine and McGregor (1993) report that one study of pregnant women suggested that only 20% of patients with TV were symptomatic. Patients who are asymptomatic may develop symptoms over a period of time.

Although symptoms vary between individuals, 50–75% of patients complain of a vaginal discharge, which may be of varying consistency, and about half of these women have a yellow-green discharge which appears frothy on examination (Heine & McGregor, 1993). Rein and Müller (1990) note that a smelly discharge is more likely to be found with BV, though a few patients with TV have a discharge with an odour. They also suggest that 25–50% of patients with TV have pruritus, which may be severe, and dyspareunia is found in up to 50% of infected women, though dysuria and frequency are generally mild and appear like cystitis.

Csonka (1990b) notes that symptoms may be worse during or following menstruation and also during pregnancy. Rein and Müller (1990) feel that although lower abdominal pain may be present in a few women, other STDs may be the cause and should be investigated.

Erythema of the vagina is present in 20–75% of women and the vaginal walls may appear granular in severe cases (Rein & Müller, 1990). Csonka (1990b) notes that vulval and perivulval erythema and oedema with excoriated skin may be present in severe infection. Pinpoint bleeding showing on the vaginal wall and cervix as red spots is described as a strawberry appearance. This is only seen in 1–2% of patients when examined by the naked eye, though it is seen in up to 42% on colposcopic examination (Wølner-Hanssen et al., 1989). Although finding a strawberry cervix is highly suggestive of TV infection, some women have no inflammation at all (Rein & Müller, 1990).

THE LIBRARY
KENT ... ORITAL
T... ...
KENT TN ...

Diagnosis in women

There are several methods of diagnosis available, though the use of clinical findings alone may be inaccurate due to the variation in signs and symptoms between patients.

Microscopy of wet slides

Lossick and Kent (1991) state that wet mount of vaginal discharge has been in use for 150 years for diagnosing TV and it is probably the most widely used method of diagnosis. The advantages of wet mount or wet prep slides are that it is relatively easy to perform and it can be carried out in the clinical area, giving immediate results. Although the test is 100% reliable if motile organisms are found, the sensitivity may be lower if the test is not performed by a skilled microscopist. Lossick and Kent (1991) found that 60–92% of infections may be found by a highly trained researcher, but only 45–60% by an average microscopist.

A specimen is taken from the posterior fornix as described in Chapter 1 and is then examined under the microscope, using either reduced or dark field illumination (Csonka, 1990b). Diagnosis is through identifying TV by its characteristic jerky movements, undulating membrane and beating flagellae. The more organisms present, the easier it is to make a positive diagnosis, but if one organism is identified then a positive diagnosis is given (Rein & Müller, 1990).

Stained slides

TV may be picked up on cervical cytology smears, and an experienced cytologist will diagnose similar amounts of infection as with the use of wet prep slides, with a specificity of 99% (Lossick & Kent, 1991). However, Petersen et al. (1995) suggest that if TV is found on cytology, a culture and wet prep should be repeated.

Gram staining is not recommended, as it is difficult to differentiate TV from pus cells using this method (Rein & Müller, 1990).

Culture

Various culture media are available for the diagnosis of TV. Generally, specimens are kept incubated for 48 hours and then examined daily for trichomonads for up to 7 days (Rein & Müller, 1990). Using culture media encourages proliferation of TV from the original specimen and a high degree of sensitivity (92–95%) is obtained by culture (Lossick & Kent, 1991). However, culture takes longer and costs more than wet prep.

Other tests

Lossick and Kent (1991) note that direct enzyme immunoassay and direct immunofluorescence assay have both been used to diagnose TV. However, sensitivities for these methods are only available from research data rather than from actual use of these techniques in a laboratory. They also suggest that the latex agglutination test may be of use as an alternative to wet prep, but it has not been fully examined or marketed.

Clinical features in men

Most men with trichomoniasis are asymptomatic and they often present at clinics as contacts of women with TV (Rein & Müller, 1990). Csonka (1990b) suggests that TV will only be found in 30–40% of male contacts and even less if sexual contact was 2 weeks or more previously.

Although TV may cause non-gonococcal urethritis (NGU), Adler (1990) believes it is an uncommon cause of urethral discharge in men and, if present, discharge may be in small amounts, sometimes only first thing in the morning before urine is passed. It has been found that men may complain of a purulent discharge, dysuria and pruritus. Rein and Müller (1990) suggest that in men, TV urethritis seems to be self-limiting.

Diagnosis in men

Although it is fairly routine to do a wet prep on female patients in GUM, it is not routine practice to actively look for TV in men, and Rein and Müller (1990) believe it can be difficult to find TV in urine or discharge from men. Saxena and Jenkins (1991) found that men who are at risk of other STDs may have TV and many more cases are found when multiple diagnostic tests are used. Specimens for TV are usually only taken from men who are sexual contacts of women known to have TV, or men who have not responded to conventional therapy for NGU (Adler, 1990).

A wet prep from the urethra is examined in the same way as for women. The two-glass urine test can also be used to diagnose TV, if the urine in the first glass is centrifuged and the sediment examined by microscopy and culture (Saxena & Jenkins, 1991), although this method is not often used.

Attempts at isolating TV from a urethral smear are often unsuccessful, possibly due to the washing or flushing away of the organism during urination or because TV do not grow easily in the environment found in the male urethra (Csonka, 1990b) and therefore only transient infection is produced.

Treatment

Metronidazole is the most widely used drug in the treatment of trichomoniasis. Csonka (1990b) suggests 200 mg of metronidazole three times a day for 7 days and notes that it usually cures 90% of cases of TV infection. Alternatively, a single dose of 2 g of metronidazole may be given to improve patient compliance (Rein & Müller, 1990); Heine and McGregor (1993) suggest the use of metronidazole by vaginal pessary or gel at the same time as single dose treatment. As metronidazole is usually avoided during early pregnancy, clotrimazole pessaries 100 mg for six nights may be used, though the cure rate may be only 50% (Csonka, 1990b).

There have been incidences of resistance to metronidazole in patients with trichomoniasis, though usually this can be overcome by altering the dosage (Heine & McGregor, 1993). In addition, it is very important that patients are advised of the side effects of metronidazole as described earlier.

Follow-up

Patients should be advised not to have sexual intercourse until they have returned to the GUM clinic for a test of cure, generally after a week, to ensure that the infection has been treated successfully. Contact slips should be given and contacts encouraged to attend. Most researchers believe that male contacts of women with TV should be treated epidemiologically, even if there are no symptoms (Rein & Müller, 1990), and as TV is often associated with other STDs, sexual contacts should have a full screen to exclude other infection (Csonka, 1990b).

In many GUM clinics, nurses manage the follow-up of patients with trichomoniasis and the authors suggest the following regimen. Women with TV should be seen after a week for a test of cure, and as a high percentage of patients have concomitant infection it is important to check that other diagnostic tests carried out at the initial visit, such as gonorrhoea cultures, are negative. A wet and dry slide should be taken for test of cure and if TV is diagnosed or the patient has symptoms, she should be managed following the clinic protocol, which may involve the patient being referred to the medical staff, though protocols vary from clinic to clinic.

Men should return after a week to have an early morning smear taken, and a wet and dry slide should be taken for direct microscopy. If both are negative, the patient should be asked to return for further follow-up if symptoms recur. Positive results should be managed as the clinic protocol directs.

Preventing recurrence

It appears that the body does not develop any immunity to TV to prevent repeated infection (Rein & Müller, 1990). It is important therefore to discuss prevention of re-infection with patients, so that they can make informed choices about their sexual health. Patients should be encouraged to be aware of their own bodies, for example, to consider not having sex if they have a discharge and to use barrier methods of contraception such as condoms and the diaphragm.

It may be helpful to introduce the idea of using the female condom, as one study has shown that using this method can effectively reduce recurrent vaginal trichomoniasis (Soper et al., 1993).

Implications for nursing practice

The three most common conditions associated with vaginal discharge have been discussed in this chapter. It has been estimated that 20–25% of women will suffer from vaginal discharge at some stage in their lives and it is important that nurses in GUM are able to distinguish between normal and abnormal vaginal discharge. Table 7.2 compares clinical features and tests for BV, candidiasis and TV.

Nursing staff in many sexual health care settings are responsible for the patient's management at the follow-up visit, including interviewing, performing follow-up examinations and giving results to the patient. This presents an ideal opportunity for health promotion, though it does have implications for professional practice. Therefore, nurses must be competent in their own practice, well trained, experienced and up-to-date with new developments.

Table 7.2: Table of signs, symptoms and tests for differential diagnosis

	Normal	Bacterial vaginosis	Candidiasis	Trichomoniasis
Symptoms	None, physiological	Offensive smell, worsens after coitus or menses	Vulval itching, discharge, irritation, dyspareunia, worsens after menses	Profuse purulent discharge, offensive smell, dyspareunia, worsens after menses
Signs	Variable clear/white discharge	Moderate white/grey homogeneous discharge, offensive odour, no local inflammation	Inflammation of labia, vulva and vagina Moderate adherent white discharge	Excessive yellow-green frothy discharge Inflammation of vulval and vaginal epithelium
pH	4.2–4.5	>4.5	>4.5	>4.5
Amine test	Negative	Positive	Negative	+ / -
Microscopy	Lactobacilli	Clue cells	Pseudomycelia, spores	Motile trichomonads
Culture	Not done	Not done	Useful for confirmation in recurrent cases	Useful if facilities permit
GU screen	Offer screen if change in recent partner	Offer screen to exclude other causes	Offer screen if change in partner	Screen for gonorrhoea and chlamydia

References

Adler MW (1990) ABC of Sexually Transmitted Diseases, 2nd edn. London: British Medical Association.

Ahmed-Jushuf IH, Shahmanesh M, Arya OP (1995) The treatment of bacterial vaginosis with a 3 day course of 2% clindamycin cream: results of a multicentre, double blind, placebo controlled trial. Genitourinary Medicine 71(4): 254–6.

Amsel R, Totten PA, Spiegel CA, Chen KCS, Eschenbach D, Holmes KK (1983) Nonspecific vaginitis: diagnostic criteria and microbial and epidemiologic associations. The American Journal of Medicine 74:14–22.

Boeke AJP, Dekker JH, Van Eijk JTM, Kostense PJ, Bezemer PD (1993) Effect of lactic acid suppositories compared with oral metronidazole and placebo in bacterial vaginosis: a randomised clinical trial. Genitourinary Medicine 69(5): 388–92.

Bowman C (1993) Recurrent bacterial vaginosis. British Journal of Sexual Medicine (Jan/Feb): 24–5.

Brand JM, Galask RP (1986) Trimethylamine: the substance mainly responsible for the fishy odor often associated with bacterial vaginosis. Obstetrics and Gynecology 68(5): 682–5.

Brockhurst P, Mindel A (1993) Recurrent genital infections. British Journal of Sexual Medicine Compendium: 24–7.

Conway M, Humphries E (1994) Bernhard Clinic meeting need in lesbian sexual health care. Nursing Times 90(32): 40–1.

Cook RL, Redondo-Lopez V, Schmitt C, Meriwether C, Sobel JD (1992) Clinical, microbiological, and biochemical factors in recurrent bacterial vaginosis. Journal of Clinical Microbiology 30(4): 870–7.

Csonka GW (1990a) Genital candidiasis. In Csonka GW, Oates JK (Eds), Sexually Transmitted Diseases – A Textbook of Genitourinary Medicine. London: Baillière Tindall.

Csonka GW (1990b) Trichomonas vaginalis infestation. In Csonka GW, Oates JK (Eds), Sexually Transmitted Diseases – A Textbook of Genitourinary Medicine. London: Baillière Tindall.

Dawson S (1990) Bacterial vaginosis. In: Csonka GW, Oates JK (Eds), Sexually Transmitted Diseases – A Textbook of Genitourinary Medicine. London: Baillière Tindall.

Dhar J, Arya OP, Timmins DJ, Moss S, Mukembo S, Alawattegama AB, Williams O (1994) Treatment of bacterial vaginosis with a three day course of 2% clindamycin vaginal cream: a pilot study. Genitourinary Medicine 70(2): 121–3.

Dockerty WG, Sonnex C (1995) Candidal balano-posthitis: a study of diagnostic methods. Genitourinary Medicine 71(6): 407–9.

Easmon CSF, Hay PE, Ison CA (1992) Bacterial vaginosis: a diagnostic approach. Genitourinary Medicine 68(2): 134–8.

Eschenbach DA (1993) History and review of bacterial vaginosis. American Journal of Obstetrics and Gynecology 169(2): 441–5.

Eschenbach DA, Hillier S, Critchlow C, Stevens C, Derouen T, Holmes KK (1988) Diagnosis and clinical manifestations of bacterial vaginosis. American Journal of Obstetrics and Gynecology 158(4): 819–27.

Fong IW (1992) The value of chronic suppressive therapy with itraconazole versus clotrimazole in women with recurrent vaginal candidiasis. Genitourinary Medicine 68(6): 374–7.

Fong IW, Bannatyne RM, Wong P (1993) Lack of in vitro resistance of *Candida albicans* to ketoconazole, itraconazole and clotrimazole in women treated for recurrent vaginal candidiasis. Genitourinary Medicine 69(1): 44–6.

Gardner HL, Dukes CD (1955) *Haemophilus vaginalis* vaginitis. American Journal of Obstetrics and Gynecology 69(5): 962–76.

Geiger AM, Foxman B, Sobel JD (1995) Chronic vulvovaginal candidiasis: characteristics of women with *Candida albicans*, C glabrota and no candida. Genitourinary Medicine 71(5): 304–7.

Gibbs RS (1993) Chorioamnionitis and bacterial vaginosis. American Journal of Obstetrics and Gynecology 169(2): 460–2.

Godley MJ (1993) The management of sexually transmitted diseases in pregnancy. Medicine International 21(3): 74–81.

Heine P, McGregor JA (1993) *Trichomonas vaginalis*: a reemerging pathogen. Clinical Obstetrics and Gynecology 36(1): 137–44.

Hill GB (1993) The microbiology of bacterial vaginosis. American Journal of Obstetrics and Gynecology 169(2): 450–4.

Hopkins SJ (1992) Drugs and Pharmacology for Nurses, 11th edn. Edinburgh: Churchill Livingstone.

Ison CA, Taylor RFH, Link C, Buckett P, Harris JRW, Easmon CSF (1987) Local treatment for bacterial vaginosis. British Medical Journal 295: 886.

Kennedy R (1995) Causes and diagnosis. British Journal of Sexual Medicine Supplement 22: 5–7.

Larsson P-G, Platz-Christensen J-J, Sundström E (1991) Is bacterial vaginosis a sexually transmitted disease? International Journal of STD & AIDS 2: 362–4.

Lossick JG (1990) Treatment of sexually transmitted vaginosis/vaginitis. Review of Infectious Diseases 12(6): S665–81.

Lossick JG, Kent HL (1991) Trichomoniasis: trends in diagnosis and management. American Journal of Obstetrics and Gynecology 164(4): 1217–22.

McGregor JA, French JI, Seo K (1993) Premature rupture of membranes and bacterial vaginosis. American Journal of Obstetrics and Gynecology 169(2): 463–6.

Moi H, Erkkola R, Jerve F, Nelleman G, Bymose B, Alaksen K, Tornqvist E (1989) Should male consorts of women with bacterial vaginosis be treated? Genitourinary Medicine 65: 263–8.

Nayagam AT, Smith MD, Ridgway GL, Allason-Jones E, Robinson AJ, Stock J (1992) Comparison of ofloxacin and metronidazole for the treatment of bacterial vaginosis. International Journal of STD & AIDS 3: 204–7.

Peel KR, MacLean AB (1995) Benign and malignant disorders of the vagina. In Whitfield CR (Ed.), Dewhurst's Textbook of Obstetrics and Gynaecology for Postgraduates, 5th edn. Oxford: Blackwell Science.

Petersen CS, Carl L, Alnor D, Thomsen U, Thomsen HK (1995) Ignored trichomonal infestation diagnosed by Papanicolaou smear. International Journal of STD & AIDS 71(4): 257–8.

Rashid S, Collins M, Kennedy RJ (1991) A study of candidosis: the role of fomites. Genitourinary Medicine 67: 137–42.

Rein MF (1990) Vulvovaginitis and cervicitis. In Mandell GL, Douglas (Jr) RG,

Bennett JE (Eds), Principles and Practice of Infectious Diseases, 3rd edn. New York: Churchill Livingstone.

Rein MF, Müller M (1990) *Trichomonas vaginalis* and trichomoniasis. In Holmes KK, Mårdh P-A, Sparling PF, Weisner PJ (Eds), Sexually Transmitted Diseases, 2nd edn. New York: McGraw-Hill.

Robertson DHH, McMillan A, Young H (1989) Clinical Practice in Sexually Transmissable Diseases, 2nd edn. Edinburgh: Churchill Livingstone.

Sanz FS, Hernanz ADP (1987) Randomized comparative trial of three regimens of itraconazole for treatment of vaginal mycoses. Review of Infectious Diseases 9: S139–42.

Saxena SB, Jenkins RR (1991) Prevalence of *Trichomonas vaginalis* in men at high risk for sexually transmitted diseases. Sexually Transmitted Diseases 18(3): 138–42.

Schnell JD (1982) Investigations into the pathoaetiology and diagnosis of vaginal mycoses. Chemotherapy 28: 14–21.

Sobel JD (1986) Recurrent vulvovaginal candidiasis. The New England Journal of Medicine 315(23): 1455–8.

Soper DE, Shoupe D, Shangold GA, Shangold MM, Gutmann J, Mercer L (1993) Prevention of vaginal trichomoniasis by compliant use of the female condom. Sexually Transmitted Diseases 29(3): 137–9.

Tobin JM, Loo P, Granger SE (1992) Treatment of vaginal candidosis: a comparative study of the efficacy and acceptability of itraconazole and clotrimazole. Genitourinary Medicine 68: 36–8.

Turner P, Richens A (1978) Clinical Pharmacology, 3rd edn. Edinburgh: Churchill Livingstone.

Upjohn (1992) Cleocin®. Drug information leaflet. Kalamazoo: Upjohn.

Wølner-Hanssen P, Krieger JN, Stevens CE, Kiviat NB, Koutsky L, Critchlow C, DeRouen T, Hillier S, Holmes KK (1989) Clinical manifestations of vaginal trichomoniasis. JAMA 261(4): 571–6.

Woolley P (1994) Diagnosis and management of vaginal infections. Part 2. British Journal of Sexual Medicine (May/June): 16–18.

Woolley P (1995a) Vulvovaginal candidosis. British Journal of Sexual Medicine Supplement 22: 4.

Woolley P (1995b) Recurrent disease. British Journal of Sexual Medicine Supplement 22: 8–10.

Chapter 8
Genital warts

Paul Husband

Introduction

Genital wart virus infection is one of the most common conditions encountered in genito-urinary medicine (GUM) clinics in Great Britain, with 49 052 first infections and 37 673 recurrent infections seen in GUM in 1994 (DOH, 1995). For many nurses working within GUM, the assessment and treatment of warts, following initial diagnosis and prescription of treatment by a doctor, can account for a large percentage of their working time. In addition, many patients are likely to suffer numerous ongoing recurrences of the problem, leading to the need for emotional support from the nurse as well as physical treatment of the warts themselves. When the likelihood of recurrence is added to the very real physical pain caused by some of the treatments, one can soon begin to appreciate that, although genital warts are considered to be one of the more minor conditions treated in GUM departments across the country, a very broad range of skills is needed to deal with this problem in its entirety and in a holistic manner.

History

Genital warts, or condylomata acuminata, were first identified several centuries ago and were originally thought to be one of the manifestations of syphilis (Oriel, 1990). Later, they were thought to be due to gonorrhoea and then to genital irritation. It had long been thought that warts were infectious, but it was not until 1954 that a study of vulval warts among the wives of soldiers returning from the Far East confirmed this (Barrett, Silbar & McGinley, 1954). It was also in the middle years of this century that the causative agent was finally identified – the human papilloma virus (HPV). In the years since this discovery, over 50 HPV types have been isolated (Oriel & Walker, 1990).

Aetiology

Genital warts, just like ordinary skin warts and veruccae, are epidermal tumours caused by papillomaviruses. The strains of HPV that cause genital warts are closely related to those that cause both skin warts and veruccae. Certain types of HPV are more strongly implicated in the development of warts than others, while other types are seen as being more likely to lead to problems such as cervical intraepithelial neoplasia (CIN) and carcinoma of the cervix, which is covered more fully in Chapter 2.

Shah (1990) states that 'the initial event in wart formation is very probably trauma to the epithelium and the entry of the virus into one or a few cells of the basal germinal layer'. The papilloma viruses then multiply inside the nuclei of the basal cells, as they are the only cells in the epithelium that are capable of dividing. Cells from all layers of the normal epithelium are found in the wart itself, thus reinforcing the fact that the wart is a tumour of the epidermis. Warts often retain normal skin coloration, but may show hyperkeratosis, hyperplasia or overgrowth of the horny layers of the skin.

'Each genital HPV type infects certain sites preferentially and produces a defined spectrum of pathological effects' (Shah, 1990). Three of the most common HPV types isolated from the genital tract of both males and females, are types 6, 11 and 16. Each of these can cause asymptomatic infection in equal proportions, flat condylomata or large, raised (exophytic) warts. HPV type 6 is four times more likely to cause exophytic warts than HPV type 16. Each of the types 6, 11 and 16 are equally likely to be present in low-grade CIN, although HPV type 16 is two to three times more likely to show up in high-grade CIN and over three times more likely to be found in invasive cervical carcinomas (Shah, 1990).

Pathogenesis

As with many other viral agents, wart virus can be present in the body without ever causing any clinical symptoms (Oriel, 1990). Daniels and Harvey (undated) suggest that up to 50% of women with HPV are asymptomatic. However, in the GUM department, patients with symptomatic infections tend to be seen, i.e. they have come along to the clinic because they have warts. With the increasing emphasis on contact tracing or partner notification, this picture is gradually changing, as more asymptomatic partners attend for routine screening.

Incidence

It has been estimated that approximately 77 000 people in the UK are affected by genital warts each year (Daniels & Harvey, undated) and about 60% of sexual partners who have contact with symptomatically infected people will go on to acquire the infection themselves, normally within 3 months (Oriel & Walker, 1990; Daniels & Harvey, undated). Thus, it is easy to see why the diagnosis and treatment of wart virus infection makes up such a large part of the workload in GUM, constituting about 12% of all infections treated. Genital warts are the most common viral sexually transmitted disease (STD) seen in GUM departments today, occurring three times more often than genital herpes (DOH , 1995).

It has long been recognised that the majority of patients suffering from a first attack of genital warts are young adults in the 20–24 year age group (King, Nicol & Rodin, 1980; Robertson, McMillan & Young, 1989; Oriel & Walker, 1990) with the most common age of onset being 22 years for men and 19 years for women. The factor that patients of all ages find most disconcerting is the very long incubation period associated with wart virus infections, which can vary between 3 weeks and 8 months. The average time between infection and manifestation is about 3 months (Robertson, McMillan & Young, 1989), though some patients would lead you to suspect an even longer period than this. The sudden appearance of a first attack of warts in an unsuspecting partner can have a very disruptive effect upon a relationship, even though in reality it does not automatically suggest infidelity. Inside a relationship, it may provoke many questions and the nurse can often play a major role in diffusing a difficult situation for both partners by answering these questions truthfully and realistically.

Another aspect of wart virus infection that many patients have difficulty understanding is why only 60% of sexual partners become infected. Why do they have warts when their one and only partner is free of them? The same reason applies as for other conditions such as influenza and the common cold: an infection does not automatically develop because one has had contact with it, because everyone has differing levels of immunity to certain viruses at different times. The author has found that many patients attending GUM clinics find it useful to sit and chat for a while about immunity: how it can prevent some people from picking up the virus in the first place, how it can prevent others from having symptoms although they have acquired the virus and how it will eventually regain control over the virus, even in those people who have had numerous recurrences. Oriel & Walker (1990) note that actual scientific knowledge about immunological response to wart virus infection is quite sparse, though Shah (1990) suggests that when the immune system is lowered, for example by pregnancy or transplantation, HPV infection is more prevalent.

An individual practitioner may not be able to advise patients on any or all of these areas, but just taking the time to talk about them can often be beneficial. It can also be helpful to establish whether either the index patient or a partner, be it past or present, has had warts on the hands, as auto-inoculation with virus from warts on the hands has been implicated in the development of genital warts (King, Nicol & Rodin, 1980).

Associated infections

An important point to be remembered by both nursing and medical staff is that many people with genital warts have other infections at the same time, so routine screening for other STDs should always be carried out at the time of the first attendance. One study showed that in men with penile warts, 10% also had gonorrhoea and another 17% had non-gonococcal urethritis (NGU), and in female attenders with warts, there was a 12% likelihood of gonorrhoea and a 12% chance of trichomoniasis (TV) being found (Kinghorn, 1978). Concurrent infection with gonorrhoea, NGU, chlamydia or TV has also been noted by Oriel and Walker (1990).

Clinical signs and symptoms

The clinical manifestations of HPV infection are varied and widespread. Any parts of the male and female genitalia can be affected, though it is more commonly seen on the moister areas and usually starts where one is more susceptible to trauma during sexual intercourse (Oriel, 1990; Oriel & Walker, 1990). Moisture as a result of concomitant infection, perspiration or poor personal hygiene at this site then provides good conditions for the warts to flourish (King, Nicol & Rodin, 1980).

Warts can be found around the anus or in the anal canal. When warts appear around the anus, it is necessary to perform a proctoscopy examination to be sure of the extent of the disease (Oriel & Walker, 1990). Condylomata acuminata can also develop on the lip or in the mouth after orogenital contact with an infected person (Oriel & Walker, 1990; Daniels & Harvey, undated). Examples of how warts may present are shown in the photographs.

Men

Soft, fleshy and vascular (exophytic) condylomas can appear in any part of the genital area, most commonly the glans penis, frenum, coronal sulcus and lining of the prepuce, as distinct from the flatter, more papular warts that appear mainly on the shaft of the penis, which is a dry area. The flatter, more papular warts are often very similar to plane warts on other non-genital areas of the skin (Oriel, 1990). Warts on the scrotum are less common (King, Nicol & Rodin, 1980).

Oriel and Walker (1990) note that about 5% of men with genital warts have urethral condylomata and that while many men are asymptomatic, some do give a history of urethral discharge or bleeding, dysuria or a poor urinary stream. The virus can spread to any part of the urethra but it rarely affects the bladder (Oriel, 1990).

Women

The areas of the female genital tract that are most commonly affected are discussed by Oriel (1990), who states that the fourchette and labia are the areas where warts normally appear first; spread to the vulva is often seen very quickly. Condylomas on the perineum and peri-anal area are seen in about 20% of cases and there may be warts in the vagina (Oriel,1990). He also notes that flat, papular warts may appear on the labia and perineum.

Warts can become quite extensive and vascular during pregnancy (Brunham, Holmes & Embree, 1990), but often they disappear completely or are more responsive to treatment after delivery (Oriel & Walker, 1990).

More than 50% of women with vulval warts show evidence of cervical HPV disease on cytology and/or colposcopy examination (Oriel & Walker, 1990). In fact, HPV on the cervix is one of the commonest causes for abnormal smear tests (Daniels & Harvey, undated).

Children

Genital warts can occur in children as well as adults (Sait & Garg, 1985) and tend to affect girls more than boys (Stumpf, 1980). It is possible that the virus may be transmitted by close physical contact with an infected person or by vertical transmission, but the risk of sexual abuse has to be considered (Oranje et al., 1990; Williams, Srinivasan & Shanmugasundararaj, 1990).

De Jong, Weiss and Brent (1982) suggest that neonatal exposure to HPV probably occurs during birth, but Oriel (1990) states that the actual risk is not known. However, over 50% of mothers whose babies develop laryngeal papillomas have a history of condylomata acuminata (Brunham, Holmes & Embree, 1990).

Diagnosis

Both sexes are equally likely to have subclinical infection with HPV, either as well as or instead of actual warts. The fact that many areas of warty tissue are easy to diagnose clinically has been identified over the years (Oriel, 1990; Daniels & Harvey, undated), but areas which are not so clear-cut should be investigated fully. Many men attending GUM departments are worried about the presence of tiny raised sebaceous glands, known as Fordyce's spots, that are often seen in the coronal sulcus of the penis or on the inner and outer side of the prepuce. These can easily be recognised by an experienced eye and the patient's mind put at rest (Oriel, 1990). Similarly, Oriel (1990) notes that many women worry about epithelial papillae and seba-ceous glands on their vulvas and can be reassured that this is normal anatomy. Experience and training are often the only way a practi-tioner can decide whether a wart that has been treated has actually disappeared, because of the minor changes in the skin surface and texture that persist after treatment (Robertson, McMillan & Young, 1989). Molluscum contagiosum is another condition that is often mistaken for genital warts, though their hard, umbilicated surface appearance aids differential diagnosis (Oriel, 1990).

Tests are available to assist in making a diagnosis of warts and these can be performed by nurses as well as by doctors. If an area of epithelium is raised and looks suspicious, or even in the absence of any such area at the time of investigation, then the acetowhite test using 3–5% acetic acid can be used. A small amount of the solution is painted on to the area in question and it highlights any warty cells by showing up irregularity of the surface texture under magnification from a colposcope (Oriel, 1990; Soutter, 1993).

Progression

As noted previously, warts are epidermal tumours and as such they tend to spread. The speed and extent of this spread varies greatly from one individual to another and is mediated by the person's own immune response, amongst other factors. Some patients first notice their infection by the presence of one tiny wart, which, however long it is left to its own devices, remains exactly the same, becoming neither larger nor smaller. Yet, in another individual, the wart may grow into a large pedunculated wart obscuring the urinary meatus. In another patient, the wart could spread to cover more or less the whole of the prepuce or glans, with the upper surface a mass of warts raised perhaps a quarter to a third of an inch above the surface of the surrounding skin. In a female patient, one wart may spread to cover the labia and further to the perineum and anus. Spontaneous halt of spread may also occur, as may spontaneous regression without treatment.

As this progression/regression appears to be controlled by the patient's own immune response, any condition that affects this response can have an important influence on the state of the warts. Two conditions that should be mentioned are pregnancy and the human immunodeficiency virus (HIV), which both lessen the patient's ability to control the wart virus. It has been known for a long time that pregnancy dampens the immune response and therefore makes the immune system less efficient when faced with a number of different infections. Thus, the pregnant woman is both more likely to pick up the virus from a sexual partner and more likely to suffer a florid attack of warts. Brunham, Holmes and Embree (1990) note that warts are of concern in pregnancy for three reasons:

1.   they may enlarge and very occasionally mechanically obstruct labour;
2.   podophyllin, the most common form of treatment, is contraindicated in pregnancy;
3.   perinatal exposure to wart virus may cause laryngeal or genital papillomatosis in the infant.

Currently, caesarean section is not generally recommended to prevent exposure to the virus, but the use of treatments other than podophyllin to remove the warts before delivery is advised (Brunham, Holmes & Embree, 1990).

The progression of HIV disease, with its attendant damage to the immune system, causes the same increased likelihood of picking up the virus in the first place and the same stronger possibility of florid attacks.

A rare complication of genital warts is the giant condylomata acuminata (Buschke-Loewenstein tumour), which affects the penis and occasionally the vulva or anus (King, Nicol & Rodin, 1980; Oriel & Walker, 1990). Essentially, the giant condyloma appears to be a benign tumour, though Oriel & Walker (1990) note reports of some late malignant changes.

Information giving

Any patient who has a diagnosis of warts made during his or her attendance at the GUM clinic will need much support and information and this will be provided by all of the health care team, though perhaps the nurse has the best opportunity to provide it. GUM nurses are in the frontline in most clinics carrying out treatments for genital warts and with the development of *Guidelines for Good Practice* (GUNA, 1995a), it is to be hoped that clinics where this does not happen will review their current policies.

Doctors in GUM are often under pressure from time constraints and the numbers of patients attending, so it falls on nurses to provide information to the patients, either at the initial or subsequent attendance. Whilst giving treatment and while the patient is recovering for a few moments afterwards is an opportune and appropriate time for the nurse to provide relevant information about spread and progression of HPV, safer sex, condom use, partner notification, colposcopy, and CIN – all important areas in which patients need information and advice. Many questions arise during this intimate period of treatment, questions that many patients feel much more comfortable discussing with a nurse rather than a doctor. Many patients are worried that they are passing the virus backwards and forwards between themselves and their partner(s). Some patients do not understand the full significance of wart virus and its relation to CIN, or the importance of regular cervical cytology and/or colposcopy. Others are unclear about the use or purpose of condoms in wart virus infection or may be unsure of why contact tracing is necessary. All these questions and issues are ideally addressed by the nurse and are considered below.

Do partners pass HPV back and forth?

Many people are convinced that this must happen. If the male partner attends the GUM department for treatment and his prepuce and
penile shaft are peppered with warts while his female partner has not
developed any warts since her last attendance 3 weeks previously,
should they abandon penetrative intercourse or should they use
condoms? Will these measures prevent the woman from getting
another attack? The answers may be seen clearly when two facts are
considered:

1.   Warts are caused by HPV and as with other viruses, once
     HPV is in the body, it is there for the rest of the person's life.
2.   The possibility of recurrence is partly governed by the
     woman's own immune response. Although some schools of
     thought suggest that it is unclear whether or not re-infection
     with the same strain of HPV brings about a recurrence (Shah,
     1990), most authorities put forward the view that this is quite
     unlikely. Abstinence or condom use would definitely be
     advised with a new partner, but within a longstanding rela-
     tionship either of these two approaches can merely add to
     levels of stress, thus reducing immunity and actually increasing
     the likelihood of recurrence. Therefore, as long as both part-
     ners are happy to resume their normal pattern of intercourse,
     clinic policy within the author's own area of practice would be
     to encourage such resumption, with the proviso that both
     should continue to be regularly checked.

What is the connection between wart virus and CIN and why is regular
cytology so important?

The first point has been covered previously and in Chapter 2 and a
brief explanation of this is vital for both female sufferers and heterosexual male wart patients with present or recent sexual partners. The
strong association between HPV infection and CIN means that all
female clinic attenders should automatically be offered routine cervical cytology (Oriel & Walker, 1990) at first or subsequent attendance
and any woman with documented wart virus infection, either clinically or on cytology, should have regular smears, ideally annually, as
in the author's own area of practice.

   Also, all current or recent sexual partners of males with documented HPV infection should be encouraged to attend for routine
screening and cytology (Oriel, 1990) and this can be aided either by

the male patient himself, or by the issue of contact slips via the nurse, doctor or health adviser.

What is the place of condoms in HPV infections?

Most studies nowadays (Oriel, 1990; Daniels & Harvey, undated) state that the only foreseeable way to prevent the spread of genital HPV infections is by the avoidance of high-risk behaviour, i.e. avoid direct contact with genital warts. It is likely that the only time viral shedding takes place is when there are warts present on the surface of the skin or epithelium. However, it is important to remember that warts may be internal and therefore not visible upon immediate examination; for example, urethral warts in a male or vaginal or cervical warts in a female. Alternatively, warts may be flat or invisible on the skin surface, only showing up with the acetowhite test. Condoms may give some protection during sexual intercourse, depending upon the site of the warts (Daniels & Harvey, 1995) and Von Krogh and Wikström (1991) suggest that all new sexual contacts use them.

Discussion of this subject can provide the ideal opportunity for a short practical teaching session by the nurse on the correct use and application of condoms. Information regarding this can be found in Chapter 3.

Preparing the patient for treatment

Perhaps the two most important pieces of information the patient should be given before any type of treatment for genital warts is undertaken are as follows:

1.   There is no treatment currently available which will definitely rid the body of the virus itself. Many patients have unrealistic expectations about a cure for their condition and it is incumbent upon the practitioner initiating the therapy to give a full explanation of the true situation. There are, however, ongoing trials of numerous drugs belonging to the interferon group which, it is hoped, will help to increase the body's own immune response to viral infections such as HPV. At present though, 'no effective antiviral therapy exists' (Von Krogh & Wikström, 1991). Only symptoms can be treated and not the cause.

2.   Any of the treatments that the patient undergoes are liable to cause at best a degree of discomfort in the affected area and at worst, severe pain.

Obviously, the area of the body involved is one that is sensitive and 'precious' to the patient. The reason why many patients seek treatment for their condition, in addition to their fears over transmission of the virus, is the fact that it disfigures the genitals – warts are not aesthetically pleasing (Robertson, McMillan & Young, 1989)! Unfortunately, the very treatments that are used to rid the patient of his or her unsightly growths can also cause a degree of disfigurement if they are used injudiciously or by the inexperienced, because all the therapies work by the physical destruction of wart cells. By implication, any treatment that destroys warts can also destroy surrounding healthy tissue, causing both pain and scarring of the genitals, though scarring is likely to subside with time. If a patient asks if any scars will be left, it is important to give an honest answer with a full explanation that every effort will be made to minimise the likelihood and extent of any scarring.

Nurse treatment policies

The following range of treatments will be discussed in the next section:

1.   podophyllin
2.   podophyllotoxin
3.   trichloroacetic acid
4.   cryotherapy
5.   electrocautery
6.   hyfrecation
7.   surgical excision.

The intention is not to give an exhaustive and all-encompassing account of the relative merits and disadvantages of each form of therapy, merely an overview of each with a brief synopsis of the history, use in clinical practice, contraindications and side effects, and the ways in which nurses can approach their use on an individual patient.

Clinic policies and protocols will obviously dictate how individual nurses can assimilate this into their own area of practice and this needs to be discussed before going into detail about the individual treatments. The protocol in most clinics would currently appear to be that any patient viewed as being a new attender, i.e. either a first-time attendance or more than 3 months having elapsed since the last

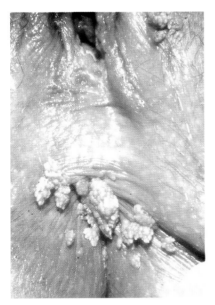

Vulval and perianal warts

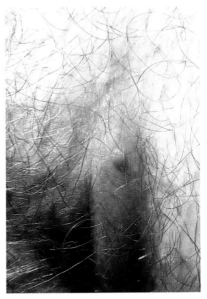

Single wart in natal cleft

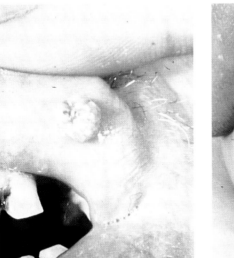

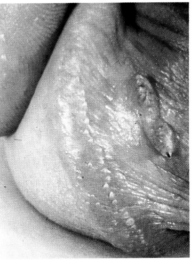

Oro-genital transmission in male homosexual partners – warts inside upper lip and on prepuce

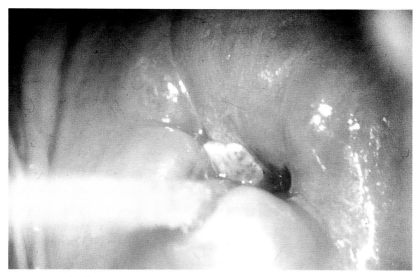

Large cervical warts

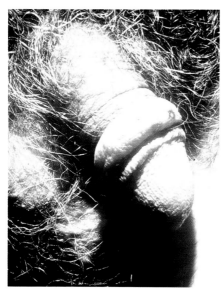

**Severe paraphimosis following
treatment with podophyllin**

attendance, will automatically be interviewed and examined by a doctor. If the presence of genital warts is noticed during this initial examination, remembering that they may or may not have been apparent to the patient beforehand, then the doctor will prescribe a course of treatment for the warts that is felt to be appropriate for the type of warts observed, for the area in which they are found and for the individual patient.

It is at this point that a great divergence of practice takes place between clinics. In some GUM departments, the doctor will apply the first treatment that he or she has prescribed and will also be responsible for reviewing the patient and the outcome of the treatment at each subsequent attendance. In other clinics, the doctor will apply the initial treatment but the patient will then be brought back for review by the nurse and for further treatment if necessary. In many clinics, the doctor prescribes the treatment for the nurse to carry out, including the initial one. It is obviously up to individual practitioners to be clear about which of these options applies in their own area of practice and to ensure that they have received appropriate training. The first of these options, in which the doctor is responsible for diagnosing, prescribing, treating and reviewing the patient throughout the whole of their care in the GUM department, allows the nurse to take very little responsibility, though it is to be hoped that this is not the case in most clinics nowadays.

It is with the other two options, which both place much more responsibility onto the nurse as an accountable practitioner, that the true worth of GUM nurses can be appreciated. This responsibility can be supported in several ways. In many GUM departments, the care plan has become an integral part of the nurses' care of patients with genital warts. Care plans often contain a detailed and accurate diagrammatic representation of the genital area of the relevant sex, upon which the nurse can document up-to-date information about the patient's current wart infection. The care plan may also provide space for a current prescription, any other advice given to the patient such as saline bathing, collateral damage from the treatment being administered, the patient's ability to tolerate the discomfort of treatment, the length of time before next suggested review and who should do this review. In those clinics where separate care plans are not the norm, these important pieces of information can be written in the medical notes.

Many clinics already follow the *Guidelines for Good Practice* (GUNA, 1995a), in that a set number of treatments are prescribed at the onset of the course and when that number has been reached, the patient is once more reviewed by a doctor, with a view to continuing with the same mode of treatment or changing to a different one. Other clinics have nurse practitioners in post, who are often able to change the prescription themselves, if necessary, in line with their clinic protocol.

However, it must be constantly borne in mind that a huge onus rests on the nurse in all of these instances. One has to be completely sure about the appearance of different kinds of warts, the advisability and necessity or otherwise of treatment for the individual at this time, the mode of action of the prescribed treatment and the response to previous treatments, as well as caring for the psychological wellbeing of the patient.

Treatment

Podophyllin

Podophyllin is a resin extracted from the roots of different species of Berberidaceae, or May Apple, and its medicinal qualities have been recognised for centuries. Over the last 50 years it has been the most commonly used treatment for genital warts (Birley, 1994).

In the author's area of clinical practice, podophyllin resin is supplied ready-to-use from the pharmacy in a 20% solution of tincture of benzoin, though 10%, 15% and 25% strengths are available on request. However, only one strength is deemed to be necessary, as a double-blind trial revealed no significant difference in outcome between 10% and 25% solutions of podophyllin (Simmons, 1981).

Podophyllin acts by destroying keratinocytes and dermal cells and by injury to the microcirculation. It is a cytotoxic agent and can cause irritation of the surrounding skin and mucous membrane, or chemical burns and painful ulceration (King, Nicol & Rodin, 1980). Great care must be taken at all times to limit the application of the liquid to the lesions themselves and any surrounding tissue, by the use of the smallest available swab or the tip of an orange-stick. Where podophyllin is used on large or extensive warts this can be quite time-consuming for the nurse, but is preferable to allowing the resin to spread over non-affected skin and mucous membrane, thereby causing unnecessary damage.

There are numerous drawbacks to the use of podophyllin. First, its efficacy and adverse effects are unpredictable (Birley, 1994). It is not a uniform substance, with the content of its active component, podophyllotoxin, varying between 2% and 10% and being relatively unstable in solution (Murphy & Bloom, 1991). Crystallisation out of solution is also common. The initial reported success rates for treatment with podophyllin were very encouraging, though more recent studies have not supported this (Gabriel & Thin, 1983; Lassus, 1987).

As previously stated, podophyllin is locally toxic, causing chemical burns and skin irritation, but it is also systemically toxic. Systemic absorption and severe neurological side effects have been noted as a result of excessive quantities of podophyllin being applied to large lesions (Oriel & Walker, 1990). Its use is also contraindicated in pregnancy because it is an antimitotic agent and it has profound effects on tissues with rapid cell division, such as the developing foetus (Murphy & Bloom, 1991). Treatment of large vascular warts with podophyllin has led to both maternal and neonatal deaths (Brunham, Holmes & Embree, 1990). Therefore, any woman of childbearing age should have a very detailed sexual history taken to rule out the possibility of pregnancy before being prescribed this particular treatment and if there is any possibility of pregnancy whatsoever, then an alternative should be used.

The most likely side effect that the nurse will observe following treatment with podophyllin, is local burning and irritation. This can be minimised by advising the patient to leave the first application in place for no longer than 4 hours (Oriel & Walker, 1990) and by allowing the podophyllin to dry fully before releasing the prepuce or closing the labia or buttocks, thus ensuring that it remains in contact only with the wart rather than other tissue. The advantage of using podophyllin is that it is easy to see just how much is being applied because of its brown colour. Chemical burns that do occur, either through over-application or abnormal susceptibility, can range from localised necrosis and ulceration at the site to more generalised redness, swelling and oedema of the genital/perianal area. Saline bathing remains the treatment of choice for reducing the severity of these unwanted side effects and is often advised prophylactically as a matter of course.

Treatments can be carried out once or twice a week for 4 weeks, at times that best suit the patient within the constraints of clinic opening-times. If the warts have not responded to treatment after 4 weeks, an alternative treatment should be considered (Oriel & Walker, 1990).

Podophyllotoxin

Podophyllotoxin is the purified active ingredient of podophyllin. It has many fewer problems than the parent drug, as it is chemically stable and present in a fixed concentration (Birley, 1994). Several studies have shown that podophyllotoxin also gives a superior therapeutic outcome to podophyllin because of its better efficacy and lower toxicity, and it is licensed for self-treatment by the patient whereas podophyllin can only be applied by a clinical practitioner (Baker et al., 1990; Murphy & Bloom, 1991; Birley, 1994).

Various companies produce 0.5% solutions of podophyllotoxin sold under trade names such as Condyline, Warticon and Warticon-Fem. Warticon-Fem has within the last 2 years been licensed for self-treatment by women, though the same advice about pregnancy holds true for this drug as with podophyllin (Birley, 1994). Each of the different brands comes in a small bottle of either 3 or 3.5 ml, along with a bunch of plastic applicators and is designed specifically for patient self-use. Warticon cream 0.15% is now licensed for use as an alternative to Warticon and Warticon-Fem solutions.

The nurse's responsibility when dealing with podophyllotoxin is not the application of the treatment itself, but to give the patient in-depth and detailed instruction on how to self-treat at home. Each of the formulations is designed to be used in the same way: one drop of liquid is applied to each wart twice a day for 3 days, then the patient has 4 days respite, to form a weekly cycle of therapy. Strong reinforcement of two salient points should be made – only one drop to each wart and a rest period for 4 days, otherwise the same localised side effects can result as with podophyllin. Thorough and regular hygiene should be encouraged, as it should during treatment with podophyllin, to keep the skin healthy and the warts softer and more susceptible to further treatment. Patients should be given a definite review date when they will be seen by either a doctor or a nurse, so that they do not go on self-treating too long when the treatment is ineffective. If the patient is brought back to be seen by the nurse at review, it is important for the nurse to be proficient at recognising the success or failure of treatment and to have the relevant information at his or her fingertips in terms of the appropriateness of continuation or change of treatment.

Trichloroacetic acid

Trichloroacetic acid (TCA) would now appear to be losing favour as a first-line treatment for genital warts, though it is still used in the author's clinic and many other GUM departments around the country.

The idea of having a concentrated acid applied to lesions on the genitals is, quite understandably, abhorrent to many people. At the time of writing, the dearth of recent references to its use would appear to back up the lay man's view, though King, Nicol and Rodin (1980) and Oriel and Walker (1990) emphasise that it can be a very effective remedy, if used correctly.

It is applied undiluted, using a pointed orange-stick or similar applicator with a small head, to small hyperkeratinised or intra-meatal warts, ensuring pinpoint accuracy and no spillage or overtreatment of the surrounding healthy skin. 'It is weakly destructive and rather painful, and numerous treatments may be required' (Oriel, 1990), but it does have its place in the treatment schedule as it is quite effective against small warts. However, its use offers no particular advantages over any other treatment regimens.

If great care is not exercised when applying TCA to genital warts, the treatment can result in severe tissue destruction, both to the patient and the operator. If it is allowed to spread over the surrounding tissues on the patient's genitals or happens to splash on to the nurse's hands, arms or face, then severe local tissue destruction can follow. A squeezy bottle of water with a tip that can be aimed carefully at the appropriate area to neutralise the acid, should be kept in each room where TCA is used as an emergency measure for use in case of spillage.

The author has found that many patients believe the axiom 'no pain, no gain'. In other words, they almost prefer to have a treatment that causes some discomfort, because they know that something is actually being done to rid them of their warts.

When carrying out prescribed treatment with TCA the onus is once more on the nurse, as an accountable practitioner, to be able to recognise success or failure of treatment, untoward events from the treatment and how to deal with them, and to have the necessary information to impart to the patient.

Cryotherapy

Strictly speaking, the term cryotherapy (cryo) actually covers three different and separate methods of dealing with genital warts, though each of the three involves freezing the warts themselves and a small area of the surrounding tissue.

Robertson, McMillan and Young (1989) note that 'the application of liquid nitrogen to discrete warts is sometimes effective'. As with the other two methods of cryotherapy, the aim is to freeze the wart until a halo of frozen skin is visible at the base. This actually denotes the formation of an ice-ball 1-2 mm larger than the diameter of the wart (Simmons, Langlet & Thin, 1981). A cotton-tipped applicator is immersed in a vacuum flask of liquid nitrogen, thereby absorbing some of the liquid into the tip. The applicator is then applied to the wart and the intense cold of -196 °C freezes the wart. This in itself has a destructive effect, as the fluid contained within the wart cells expands on freezing and breaks down the cell walls. It should, of course, be borne in mind, that the same thing also occurs in healthy, non-wart cells in the surrounding area, so pinpoint accuracy is again recommended.

The patient does suffer some pain with these methods, both while it is being carried out and more especially afterwards, leading to some authorities recommending the use of local anaesthesia (Oriel, 1990). Minor frostbite is actually caused during cryotherapy and the intense ache, like that experienced when frozen fingers are coming back to life after being exposed to freezing weather, is the feeling that the patient experiences in his or her genital area after cryotherapy. The patient should be warned of this beforehand and supported during the actual experience, though again, for many patients the 'no pain, no gain' philosophy comes into play.

The second method of freezing genital warts involves the use of a flask of liquid nitrogen with a spray head attached, along with a trigger and an interchangeable nozzle. The Cryo Jet and Fern Cryo are examples of equipment used in this method. The doctor or nurse selects the appropriately-sized nozzle for the wart or warts to be treated and then goes on to form a 1–2 mm ice-ball around the wart by spraying a fine jet of liquid nitrogen directly on to it.

Once more, extreme accuracy is needed and in this instance it is quite easy to ensure by careful selection of the nozzle and by holding the nozzle close to the wart. It is recommended that the nozzle is held half to three quarters of an inch away from the wart and the liquid nitrogen is sprayed in short bursts of 5 to 10 seconds at a time, stopping to allow the vapour to clear before giving another short burst. The overall aim is to maintain the wart in its frozen state for at least 30 seconds and some authorities maintain that two freezing cycles, for example a cycle of 30 seconds frozen, complete thawing, then another 30 seconds frozen, is the ideal for rapid resolution of the warts (Godley et al., 1987; McKenna & McMillan, 1990).

The third and final method is probably the most common in GUM practice today – the cryoprobe, which Oriel (1990) regards as 'a useful piece of equipment'. This can be operated either by nitrous oxide or carbon dioxide and in the author's area of clinical practice, the two have been evaluated side by side. Carbon dioxide is cheaper, it freezes to within 1°C of the effect of nitrous oxide and it gives off less toxic fumes when used in confined spaces.

The technique with this method is to use the appropriately sized tip or probe to freeze a ball of lubricating gel, thereby freezing the wart. Enough gel is applied, either to the wart itself or to the tip of the probe, to ensure a 1–2 mm ice-ball around the wart. Then, following the manufacturer's instructions for the use of the particular brand of cryoprobe, the tip of the probe is frozen by allowing the ingress of nitrous oxide or carbon dioxide. This freezes the tip, which freezes the gel, thus freezing the wart. Freeze the wart for 30 seconds, thaw, freeze the wart for 30 seconds again, is the regimen to be followed. Pain is an almost universal experience for patients undergoing this treatment and the same tenets apply with regard to accuracy of treatment. The nurse must be familiar with the appearance of warts and the necessity or desirability of treatment in each individual instance.

Each of the treatments mentioned above – podophyllin/ podophyllotoxin, TCA and cryotherapy – can be used either singly or jointly for each individual patient and for each individual wart. So one patient could have only podophyllin; while another could have a combination of TCA and podophyllin; another could have cryo and podophyllin; and another could have TCA only to urethral warts and cryo to perianal warts. Therefore, the nurse needs to have a clear understanding of the action of each treatment, its relevance to the particular type and location of the wart being treated and the wisdom of applying it in each particular instance. This can only be achieved through thorough training and experience.

The three remaining forms of treatment will be only briefly discussed, as they are not performed by nursing staff, though it is advisable that nurses are aware of them and able to assist with them.

Electrocautery

This involves using a probe through which an electric current is passed. The patient is earthed using an electrode plate, which makes the circuit complete, thus allowing the probe to burn away wart tissue. It is always carried out following an injection of local anaesthetic. Robertson, McMillan and Young (1989) state that its 'aim should be to coagulate the wart down to the basement membrane and cause minimal damage to the surrounding skin'. The nurse's role in this treatment will probably extend to preparing the trolley and relevant equipment, drawing up the local anaesthetic, site preparation, support for the patient during the procedure, application of dressings, provision of the relevant analgesia and explanation of follow-up, all as dictated by local policies and protocols. This form of treatment is regarded as being effective, although only practicable at certain sites, such as the labia majora, the perianal area and the shaft of the penis (Oriel, 1990), and like all the other treatments mentioned, does not preclude further recurrence of warts.

Hyfrecation

Hyfrecation is another treatment that uses an electric current. Again, it is usually applied after administration of a local anaesthetic. The electrode can be used in three different ways:

1.   in light contact with the wart. This causes dessication, whereby the cellular fluid is drawn from the wart tissue, leaving a dry crust which usually sloughs off in 7 to 10 days (GUNA, 1995b);
2.   in firm contact with the wart, coagulating it and burning it away as in electrocautery;
3.   close to the wart without actually touching it, resulting in sparking to the surface (fulguration). This limits tissue destruction to a shallow area under the spark (GUNA, 1995b).

Regardless of which way the hyfrecator is used, the nurse's role will be as for electrocautery.

Surgical excision

Surgical excision is a procedure generally carried out using scissors rather than a scalpel. It has been carried out under local anaesthetic to remove large warts that have not responded to other treatment (Daniels & Harvey, undated). McMillan and Scott (1987) describe a procedure suitable for carrying out in an outpatient department. As GUM clinics are outpatient departments, it is important that GUM nurses have some knowledge of the procedure.

The nurse will have the same role as described for electrocautery treatment, though in the author's experience, the problems with postoperative bleeding, pain and difficulty with keeping dressings in place tend to be more marked after this form of treatment than after either cautery or hyfrecation. The nurse will need to discuss these problems with the patient, so that he or she will be better prepared to face them when they almost inevitably occur.

Conclusion

It is important that nurses working within the field of GUM have a good foundation of knowledge and expertise with regard to caring for patients with genital wart infection. As many patients have been observed to have psychosexual problems because of genital warts (Von Krogh & Wikström, 1991), it is vital that the service given deals not only with the physical conditions with which patients present, but also with their psychosexual wellbeing. GUM nurses frequently perform expanded roles when caring for patients with HPV, while at the same time providing a large proportion of the care for such patients. It is therefore vital that every nurse in GUM is capable of giving excellent care based on knowledge and expertise.

References

Baker DA, Douglas JM, Buntin DM, Micha JP, Beutner KR, Patsner B (1990) Topical Podofilox for the treatment of condylomata acuminata in women. Obstetrics and Gynecology 76(4): 656–9.

Barrett TJ, Silbar JD, McGinley JP (1954) Genital warts – a venereal disease. JAMA 154(4): 333–4.

Birley H (1994) Podophyllotoxin a better treatment for genital warts? Journal of Sexual Health April/May: 42–5.

Brunham RC, Holmes KK, Embree JE (1990) Sexually transmitted diseases in pregnancy. In Holmes KK, Mårdh P-A, Sparling PF, Wiesner PJ (Eds), Sexually Transmitted Diseases, 2nd edn. New York: McGraw-Hill.

Daniels VG, Harvey I (undated) STD Facts, 2nd edn. Cambridge: Daniels Publishing.

De Jong AR, Weiss JC, Brent RL (1982) Condyloma acuminata in children. American Journal of Diseases in Children 136(8): 704–6.

DOH (1995) Sexually Transmitted Diseases, England 1994. Department of Health Statistical Bulletin. London: HMSO.

Gabriel G, Thin RNT (1983) Treatment of anogenital warts. Comparison of trichloroacetic acid and podophyllin versus podophyllin alone. British Journal of Venereal Diseases 59: 124–6.

Genito-Urinary Nurses Association (1995a) Wart treatments. In Guidelines for Good Practice. GUNA.

Genito-Urinary Nurses Association (1995b) Hyfrecation treatment of genital warts. GUNA News 1(1): 2.

Godley MJ, Bradbeer CS, Gellan M, Thin RNT (1987) Cryotherapy compared with trichloroacetic acid in treating genital warts. Genitourinary Medicine 63: 390–2.

King A, Nicol C, Rodin P (1980) Venereal Diseases, 4th edn. London: Baillière Tindall.

THE LIBRARY
KENT & ... SPITAL
TU... ... ELLS
KENT TN 8AT

Kinghorn GR (1978) Genital warts: incidence of associated genital infections. British Journal of Dermatology 99: 405–9.

Lassus A (1987) Comparison of podophyllotoxin and podophyllin in treatment of genital warts. Lancet: August 29: 512–13.

McKenna JG, McMillan A (1990) Management of intrameatal warts in men. International Journal of STD & AIDS 1: 259–63.

McMillan A, Scott GR (1987) Outpatient treatment of perianal warts by scissor excision. Genitourinary Medicine 63: 114–15.

Murphy M, Bloom GD (1991) Podophyllin or podophyllotoxin as treatment for condylomata acuminata? Papillomavirus Report 2(4): 87–9.

Oranje AP, De Waard-Van der Spek FB, Vuzevski VD, Bilo RAC (1990) Condylomata acuminata in children. International Journal of STD & AIDS 1: 250–5.

Oriel D (1990) Genital human papillomavirus infection. In Holmes KK, Mårdh P-A, Sparling PF, Wiesner PJ (Eds), Sexually Transmitted Diseases, 2nd edn. New York: McGraw-Hill.

Oriel JD, Walker PG (1990) Genital papilloma virus infections. In Csonka GW, Oates JK (Eds), Sexually Transmitted Diseases – A Textbook of Genitourinary Medicine. London: Baillière Tindall.

Robertson DHH, McMillan A, Young H (1989) Clinical Practice in Sexually Transmissible Diseases, 2nd edn. Edinburgh: Churchill Livingstone.

Sait MA, Garg BR (1985) Condylomata acuminata in children: report of four cases. Genitourinary Medicine 61: 338–42.

Shah KV (1990) Biology of human genital tract papillomaviruses. In Holmes KK, Mårdh P-A, Sparling PF, Wiesner PJ (Eds), Sexually Transmitted Diseases, 2nd edn. New York: McGraw-Hill.

Simmons PD (1981) Podophyllin 10% and 25% in the treatment of ano-genital warts – a comparative double-blind study. British Journal of Venereal Diseases 57: 208–9.

Simmons PD, Langlet F, Thin RNT (1981) Cryotherapy versus electrocautery in the treatment of genital warts. British Journal of Venereal Diseases 57: 273–4.

Soutter P (1993) A Practical Guide to Colposcopy. Oxford: Oxford University Press.

Stumpf PG (1980) Increasing occurrence of condylomata acuminata in premenarchal children. Obstetrics & Gynecology 56(2): 262–4.

Von Krogh G, Wikström A (1991) Efficacy of chemical and/or surgical therapy against condylomata acuminata: a retrospective evaluation. International Journal of STD & AIDS 2: 333–8.

Williams J, Srinivasan, Shanmugasundararaj A (1990) Warts on the gums in a child. International Journal of STD & AIDS 1: 136–7.

Bibliography

Allen I, Hogg D (1993) Work Roles and Responsibilities in Genitourinary Medicine Clinics. London: Policy Studies Institute.

BOC (1987) Medical gas data and safety sheet nitrous oxide, Substance Identification No. 1070. BOC Medical Gases.

BOC (1990) Medical gas data and safety sheet carbon dioxide, Substance Identification No. 1013. BOC Medical Gases.

Chapter 9
Genital herpes and molluscum contagiosum

Gabrielle McDermott

Genital herpes

Introduction

Genital *Herpes simplex* virus (HSV) infection is a disease of major public health importance, which has increased in prevalence over the last two decades. First episode genital herpes can be a severe illness while, in contrast, recurrent episodes tend to be milder and of shorter duration. However, the chronicity of recurrent disease has severe effects on personal relationships and sexuality. Transmission of the virus to babies at the time of birth is a major concern to affected women.

Studies over the last decade have shown the effectiveness and tolerance of aciclovir as an antiviral agent in reducing many of the clinical manifestations of first episodes, as well as improving the quality of life for those with frequently recurring disease. Two new antiviral agents, famciclovir (Famvir) and valaciclovir (Valtrex), are now licensed for the treatment of genital herpes and appear to be capable successors to aciclovir.

The spelling of 'acyclovir' has recently been standardised worldwide to 'aciclovir' and the latter is used in this chapter, except in references where relevant.

HSV antibodies

There are two types of HSV, type 1 and type 2. HSV type 1 is the commonest cause of herpes labialis (cold sores), which are rarely caused by type 2. HSV type 2 most commonly causes genital lesions, though genital herpes can be due to either viral type. Research carried out by Woolley and Kudesia (1990) showed that HSV type 1 was more commonly isolated from patients with first episode genital herpes than previously reported. The incidence of type 1 and type 2 isolated from women was almost equal (48% versus 52%), while in men there was a greater incidence of HSV type 2 than HSV type 1 (71% versus 29%).

Serological differentiation has, in the past, been hindered by the close antigenic similarity of the two viral types. Recently, reliable and sensitive tests have been developed in the USA to detect antibodies to HSV type 2. The seroprevalence of HSV type 2 antibody among genito-urinary medicine (GUM) clinic attenders and blood donors in London has been reported to be 22.7% in the former and 7.6% in the latter (Cowan et al., 1994). There was a strong relationship between HSV type 2 antibody and sexual lifestyle. Only a minority of those identified by serology had been diagnosed as having had clinical episodes of genital herpes.

Prevalence and transmission

Symptomatic genital herpes infection refers to clinically apparent lesions of either first episode or recurrent episode genital herpes. Lesions frequently contain high viral titres and the individual should be considered highly infectious to susceptible sexual partners. When lesions resolve, the virus is generally considered to be dormant and confined primarily to the dorsal root ganglia and the person is considered to be much less infectious (Oates, 1990). However, virus is known to be shed asymptomatically and transmission can occur in this way. Oates (1990) also notes that the frequency and duration of asymptomatic shedding and relative risk of transmission are unknown, but are likely to be small and vary between individuals.

An asymptomatic HSV infection is one that exists in a person who has no prior history of genital ulceration and who has never had any signs or symptoms to suggest that they have ever had the condition. Frequently, such people are only identified by finding asymptomatic viral shedding or serological evidence of antibody to HSV type 2, the predominantly genital strain (Corey, 1990). Asymptomatic infection can become symptomatic at any time.

Between the two extremes are people with genital lesions that may or may not recur. The lesions are atypical and, therefore, are not easily identified clinically as being due to genital herpes. These people with no apparent infection are frequently misdiagnosed as suffering from either genital trauma or recurrent thrush. Occasionally, the diagnosis is only made when specimens for virus identification prove positive during routine screening at GUM clinics.

The number of cases of genital herpes (first episode and recurrent episode) occurring annually in the UK is unknown. Reported cases from GUM clinics continue to rise and in 1994 there were 15 347 cases of first episode and 11 458 cases of recurrent episode HSV infections in England (DOH, 1995). However, there is no standard-ised reporting system for cases presenting and being treated in the community. In a survey of general practitioners (GPs), 21% treated first episodes and 47% treated recurrent episodes in the practice, without referral to a GUM clinic (Woolley & Chandiok, unpub-lished). These figures, however, are only valid for clinically apparent lesions and many atypical cases of genital infection may go unrecog-nised.

Atypical genital herpes may be an important feature in the sexual transmission of the disease. In one study, only 60% of women diag-nosed as having genital herpes by HSV culture had characteristic ulcerative lesions and many people had symptoms which neither they nor their clinician attributed to genital herpes (Koutsky et al., 1992). The prevalence of atypical presentations in the community is unknown.

HSV type 2 is most commonly acquired when a susceptible indi-vidual comes into contact with an infected person when infectious virus is present. Individual variation in susceptibility and the amount of virus present are likely to determine whether transmission takes place. Cleator and Klapper (1994) note that orogenital transmission of HSV type 1 may account for 10–40% of genital transmission. In populations in which HSV type 1 forms a large proportion of genital disease, genital to genital transmission is just as likely as orogenital transmission. Non-sexual transmission is thought to be extremely rare.

Condoms have been shown to be effective barriers to the passage of HSV (Conant, Spicer & Smith, 1984), but viral shedding may occur in areas that the condom does not cover. Spermicidal foams and creams containing nonoxynol-9 inactivate HSV. Education of patients about transmission through orogenital sex when cold sores are present, may reduce HSV type 1 transmission. However, asymp-tomatic viral shedding from the mouth will remain, albeit in small amounts. Corey (1990) considers whether genital ulceration facili-tates the spread of HIV infection in developed countries but feels that this has not yet been resolved.

Asymptomatic infection

The asymptomatic shedding of HSV may occur from macroscopically normal-looking skin or from ulcers that the person is unaware of or which are hidden, for example on the cervix or urethra. The sexual transmission of HSV in this way has been well documented and in a study of women with recurrent symptomatic genital herpes, episodes of asymptomatic shedding were documented in 14% of those cultured during asymptomatic periods (Rattray et al., 1978).

The prevalence of asymptomatic shedding and risk of transmission in patients with no previous history of genital ulceration is unknown. However, in a study of women attending a GUM clinic with first episode genital herpes whose regular male sexual partners attended, 18.3% of men had first episode genital herpes at the same time, 13.4% had signs or symptoms consistent with recurrent genital herpes and 1.8% were documented as having asymptomatic viral shedding from intact epithelium, despite no prior history of genital ulceration (Woolley, 1991).

Presentation

Patients with genital herpes may present to their GP, Accident & Emergency department or GUM clinic depending upon the severity and nature of their symptoms. Accurate diagnosis, good clinical management and early counselling are important in reducing the physical and psychological morbidity associated with the condition.

First episodes

The incubation period is generally considered to be between 2 and 12 days and the clinical features last, on average, 14 to 21 days (Cleator & Klapper, 1994). Herpetic lesions evolve from a group of pustular or vesicular papules to form discrete shallow ulcers, which frequently coalesce to form larger areas of ulceration. The ulcers then scab over and heal. However, new vesicles and ulcers may occur in crops as earlier lesions heal. Lesions are generally painful, frequently multiple and bilateral and are associated with tender inguinal lymphadenopathy. Systemic symptoms are common and include fever, myalgia (muscle pain), arthralgia (joint pain) and headache.

Lesions commonly occur on the external genitalia but can also occur in the urethra, giving rise to symptoms of urethritis with dysuria and urethral discharge or on the cervix, where they can be mistaken for a necrotic cervicitis (Oates, 1990). HSV can cause proctitis in women, due to the spread of infectious vaginal secretions and proctitis is common in homosexual men (Cleator & Klapper, 1994), where it may be associated with anorectal pain, tenesmus and constipation.

There are several important complications that may occur in the course of first episode infection. Difficulty in passing urine is a common symptom, especially in women. Occasionally, this may be due to a sacral radiculomyelopathy affecting sensory and autonomic nerves, which results in the inability to initiate micturition and is often associated with altered sensation in the perineum, thighs and buttocks (Cleator & Klapper, 1994). More commonly, there is a reflex inhibition of micturition due to the marked pain as urine flows over the ulcers (Adler, 1990). If retention of urine occurs, then catheterisation may be necessary and some clinicians favour a suprapubic approach to avoid passing infective material directly to the bladder (Oates, 1990).

Headache, photophobia and neck stiffness occurring after the eruption of genital lesions frequently indicates the occurrence of aseptic meningitis. Lumbar puncture and examination of the cerebrospinal fluid is necessary to confirm the diagnosis and exclude coexistent bacterial meningitis. The course of the condition is usually benign (Corey, 1990). Herpes encephalitis may be a serious condition that manifests as impaired consciousness, fits and the development of focal signs. The condition may progress rapidly but mortality is reduced to less than 20% if intravenous antiviral therapy is started promptly at the onset (Cleator & Klapper, 1994). The rare neurological condition of transverse myelitis has been reported (Oates, 1990), in which there is a rapid onset of symmetrical paralysis and sensory impairment of the lower limbs. Spontaneous recovery is usual, although some residual weakness may persist.

Orogenital sexual contact may be responsible for the spread of HSV to the pharynx, where it may give rise to herpetic pharyngitis. It nearly always occurs as a result of fellatio and therefore is most common in women and homosexual men (Oates, 1990). A severe sore throat and difficulty in swallowing may be indicative of first episode HSV. Signs vary from mild erythema to severe ulcerative pharyngitis.

Nursing care and management

In most cases of first episode genital herpes a clinical diagnosis can be made confidently and treatment should not be delayed until the result of confirmatory diagnostic tests are available, as symptoms often increase in the week after the lesions first develop (Corey, 1990). The individual should be informed of the likely diagnosis and be given a simple explanation of the nature of the virus and routes of transmission. Early counselling at the time of diagnosis may help address some of the fears and anxieties that patients have and it is best to back this up with up-to-date literature for the patient to take away and read at home. Adler (1990) suggests that it is important to stress the need for contact tracing and the patient should be advised to abstain from intercourse until the lesions are completely healed. Asymptomatic shedding can be discussed either at the first attendance or at a subsequent follow-up visit. Some researchers recommend the use of condoms for 3 months after resolution of the first episode, because of the increased likelihood of asymptomatic shedding during this time (Adler, 1990).

Symptomatic treatment will be required for most patients and systemic analgesia should be prescribed. Adler (1990) suggests that preferably this should be simple in nature, for example paracetamol.

Regular saline bathing (3 tablespoons of salt per bath) may give some symptomatic relief (Adler, 1990) and women should be advised to wear loose fitting undergarments to let the air circulate and help dry the lesions. Women who are experiencing pain on micturition may find it easier to pass urine while in a warm bath, which will reduce the risk of urinary retention, or occasionally, local anaesthetic gel applied 10 minutes prior to micturition may be helpful (Oates, 1990).

Oates (1990) notes that in women, there may be coinfection with *Candida albicans* and oral antifungal therapy, for example fluconazole 150 mg as a single dose or itraconazole 200 mg twice daily for one day, should be prescribed to treat this rather than topical therapy, though Corey (1990) recommends clotrimazole or nystatin. Occasionally, especially if there has been a delay in presentation, secondary bacterial infection may be present, in which case a broad spectrum antibiotic such as co-trimoxazole is recommended, as it does not mask the presence of coinfection with syphilis (Adler, 1990). However, there have been recent concerns regarding the safety of co-trimoxazole.

Specific therapy for uncomplicated first episode genital herpes is oral treatment with aciclovir 200 mg five times daily (Cleator & Klapper, 1994). Famciclovir 250 mg three times daily or valaciclovir 500 mg twice daily for 5 days have also been licensed for use. Antiviral therapy should be started as soon as possible after the onset of symptoms. Oates (1990) believes that topical therapy has little place in the management of first episodes, as although effective in reducing local symptoms and viral shedding, there is little influence on systemic symptoms and hence oral preparations are preferred. None of the above agents are licensed for use in pregnancy or during lactation.

Management of the complications of genital HSV infection will depend on the nature of the complications. Disseminated HSV infection, most commonly seen in the immunosuppressed or when first episodes occur during pregnancy, and HSV encephalitis respond best to intravenous aciclovir therapy (Cleator & Klapper, 1994).

Recurrent episodes

Many patients suffering first episodes of genital herpes will go on to experience recurrent attacks, the frequency and severity of which will vary from individual to individual. Ascent of the virus, via the sensory neurones to the dorsal root ganglia, leads to latent infection and when viral replication is stimulated the virus returns via the axons to the genital region, where it may cause clinical symptoms (Oates, 1990).

Two theories have been proposed to explain the mechanism by which HSV recurs. Corey (1990) describes them as the 'skin trigger' and the 'ganglion trigger' theories. The first theory means that the virus is continually travelling down the nerve. This would account for people who experience a recurrence soon after sexual intercourse, most commonly triggered by local trauma, and would also explain most cases of asymptomatic shedding. The second theory is that specific trigger factors act directly on the ganglia, initiating viral movement down the axons. This mechanism explains why some patients experience prodromal symptoms of itching or tingling for up to 72 hours before an attack erupts at that site. Both mechanisms probably exist in any one individual.

Following a first episode about 60% of patients with HSV type 2 will have a recurrence, but the figure for HSV type 1 is thought to be lower (Cleator & Klapper, 1994). However, the most common clinical pattern is of occasional recurrences, which decrease in frequency as the length of time since the first episode increases. Corey (1990) suggests that some patients will suffer up to five recurrences a year over the first 2 years. A minority will suffer frequent recurrences over a long period of time (Cleator & Klapper, 1994).

Recurrent genital herpes affects patients in different ways. Some may have recurrences that are so mild as to be virtually symptomless, while others suffer debilitating disease with severe prodromal symptoms and lesions that affect the genital area significantly (Oates, 1990).

The evolution of herpetic lesions through vesicle, ulcer and crusting stages is the same as in first episodes. Recurrent episodes, however, are usually well localised, well demarcated and usually last 8 to 12 days or less without treatment, as symptoms are generally less severe (Corey, 1990). Systemic upset such as fever, headache and malaise are unusual. Some patients recognise the onset of prodromal symptoms, which can be a useful marker to abstain from sexual activity, thus reducing the risk of transmission to sexual partners.

Although most people who suffer recurrences are unable to identify any precipitating factors for their attacks, a number of trigger factors have been identified, including local trauma, for example sexual intercourse; menstruation; stress; anxiety; depression; fatigue; concurrent infection; pregnancy; and ultraviolet light (Adler, 1990; Oates, 1990).

Nursing care and management

Many patients with occasional and infrequent recurrences simply require reassurance and advice about avoiding trigger factors, and guidance about managing symptoms. Measures such as saline bathing and simple analgesia will usually be sufficient (Adler, 1990).

Direct questioning about the impact of the disease on the person's lifestyle and relationships is important and may reveal problems that the individual might wish to discuss but is otherwise reluctant to volunteer. Patients may feel stigmatised by the disease or worry about infecting others, to the point of choosing celibacy (Drob, Loemer & Lifshutz, 1985). Most will be aware of the need to avoid sexual intercourse during recurrences, but it is worthwhile emphasising this point (Oates, 1990).

A man with a history of recurrent genital herpes whose partner is pregnant should be advised to use condoms or abstain from intercourse during the third trimester to avoid passing on the virus, as a woman is more susceptible to infection at this time (Woolley et al., 1988).

Women who had suffered an episode of genital herpes were, at one time, considered to be at greater risk of developing cervical intraepithelial neoplasia (CIN) and were recommended to have annual cytology. However, the risk is now thought to be much lower than previously believed and annual cytology is no longer considered necessary by many clinicians, though others still recommend it (Adler, 1990; Oates, 1990).

The Herpes Viruses Association (HVA) provides support for people suffering from herpes virus infections. Some people derive benefit from being involved in such a self-help group and may be reassured by being able to talk to people in the same situation (Adler, 1990). It is important to inform patients of this association and supply the telephone number and address, which are given at the end of this chapter.

For patients whose recurrences are frequent and/or severe, especially if the condition is causing psychological or relationship problems, episodic or continuous antiviral therapy may be prescribed. Although aciclovir cream is popular for treating mild recurrences, many physicians feel that the most effective form of episodic therapy is a five-day course of oral aciclovir 200 mg five times daily (Corey, 1990). Famciclovir 125 mg twice daily and valaciclovir 500 mg twice daily are now licensed for use in recurrent HSV and can be started at the onset of prodrome or the first local symptom.

Continuous antiviral therapy should be considered for patients who have frequent recurrences, usually eight or more attacks per year, or in any patient who is experiencing severe psychological problems because of the recurrent nature of their condition. At present, aciclovir is the only drug licensed for long-term suppression and a dose of 200 mg four times daily is given for 2 months (Oates, 1990). This dose is effective for suppression, but compliance can be a problem, leading to breakthrough recurrences. After 2 to 3 months, the dose can be reduced to the lowest possible daily dose which still achieves viral suppression (Mindel et al., 1988). Continuous suppression therapy can be given for 6 to 12 months (Oates, 1990). Both famciclovir and valaciclovir are currently in clinical trials for use as continuous therapy.

Extragenital herpes

Transfer of virus to extragenital sites at the time of first episodes can occur through auto-inoculation, particularly if personal hygiene is lacking (Oates, 1990) and such lesions can easily be misdiagnosed as recurrent shingles by GPs and patients.

Acute ocular pain, blurring of vision and excessive tear production are common symptoms of conjunctivitis and when the characteristic dendritic ulcers of HSV infection are seen, a diagnosis of herpetic keratoconjunctivitis can be made clinically and antiviral therapy initiated (Cleator & Klapper, 1994). They also note that debridement and systemic and/or topical aciclovir are valuable in achieving speedy healing of the lesions. However, the condition may recur with variable frequency and can lead ultimately to corneal scarring and loss of some visual acuity. Once recognised, a referral to an ophthalmologist is recommended.

Inoculation of the virus through a break in the skin can lead to a herpetic whitlow (Cleator & Klapper, 1994). Symptoms include the abrupt onset of oedema, erythema and localised tenderness of the infected finger. Vesicular or pustular lesions may be difficult to distinguish from bacterial infection and in both conditions, fever, lymphangitis and local lymph node enlargement may occur. Episodes usually respond well to a short course of antiviral therapy (Cleator & Klapper, 1994) but as with other sites, the condition tends to recur.

Erythema multiforme is an acute self-limiting eruption of the skin and mucous membranes, characterised by distinct target lesions of rounded erythema with central darkening – referred to as 'iris lesions' (Shelley, 1967). Cleator and Klapper (1994) note that occasionally it progresses to involve several mucosal surfaces and internal organs, accompanied by severe constitutional symptoms – 'Stevens-Johnson syndrome'. Successive crops of target lesions may appear and usually recede after 1 or 2 weeks, leaving residual hyperpigmentation. There are a number of triggers for erythema multiforme, one of which is HSV (Shelley, 1967). Recurrences are common, especially if due to recurrent episodes of HSV infection. A short course of antiviral therapy may be recommended and if recurrences are frequent and troublesome, continuous therapy should be considered (Cleator & Klapper, 1994).

Widespread lesions of HSV may occur in people with severe atopic eczema (eczema herpeticum) or who are immunosuppressed, either through drugs or disease (Cleator & Klapper, 1994). In patients with HIV/AIDS, progressive and destructive genital, perianal, perioral and extragenital lesions may occur.

Diagnosis of genital herpes

It is important that other sexually transmitted and non-sexually transmitted causes are considered in anyone presenting for the first time with genital ulceration, or if someone with known genital herpes has an atypical recurrence. Genital trauma (both accidental or self-inflicted), Behçet's disease, Crohn's disease, lichen sclerosis, lichen planus and recurrent candidiasis may be mistaken for HSV (Corey, 1990; Oates, 1990; Cleator & Klapper, 1994).

It is important to take a detailed history, noting foreign travel, recent sexual contacts and the use of barrier methods of contraception, for example condoms. All patients should have full STD screening, including dark-field microscopy and blood should be taken for syphilis serology. Serological tests should be repeated 3 months after resolution of the ulceration, as coinfection with HSV and syphilis is known (Oates, 1990).

Establishing the diagnosis of recurrent genital herpes is often straightforward, as most patients will have had a clinical and virologically confirmed first episode. However, lesions of recurrent genital herpes may be small and specimens for viral identification need to be taken as soon as possible after the onset of symptoms or lesions to confirm the diagnosis, as virus may be present for a much shorter time than in primary episodes (Corey, 1990).

Laboratory tests

It is important to confirm the diagnosis of genital herpes and there are a number of non-specific and specific tests available. Characteristic multinucleated giant cells seen on cytological examination of cervical smears or smears taken from the lesions are diagnostic of HSV infection, but the technique has a low sensitivity for detecting infected individuals (Oates, 1990). Although cytological examination is no longer used in clinical practice for the diagnosis of HSV infection, finding multinucleated giant cells on routine cervical cytological screening does indicate that the woman was shedding HSV at the time the test was performed.

Specific tests routinely available in clinical practice include HSV culture and viral antigen detection (Corey, 1990). Vesicular lesions should be carefully opened to release fluid and ulcerated lesions should be firmly rubbed with a cotton wool-tipped swab as described in Chapter 1, Appendix 1. Swabs taken from the cervix should include the ectocervix as well as the endocervical canal, as the virus predominantly affects squamous epithelium. Swabs should be transported to the laboratory in a nutrient medium containing antibiotics to suppress bacterial growth and ideally, be stored at a temperature of 4 °C (Cleator & Klapper, 1994).

HSV grows in many human and animal cell cultures and usually produces a classical cytopathic effect in 1 to 7 days (Cleator &

Klapper, 1994). Cultured virus can then be typed using anti-sera, immunofluorescence or DNA hybridisation (Oates, 1990; Cleator & Klapper, 1994). Some laboratories prefer to use techniques for viral antigen detection, either by direct immunofluorescence or enzyme-linked immunosorbent assay. The sensitivity and specificity of these tests is high, especially if used with monoclonal antibodies (Lafferty et al., 1987).

Other diagnostic tests, such as electron microscopy, are not generally available except where there is a research laboratory. Neutralising antibodies to HSV can be measured but have little use in the routine diagnosis of the condition as this method does not distinguish between the two viral types with any reliability. Serological tests using monoclonal antibodies to a glycoprotein in the HSV envelope, or using a modified Western Blot technique, have been developed with the intent of identifying those infected with HSV type 2 (Ashley et al., 1988).

Psychological response to genital herpes

Adler (1990) notes that anxiety, depression and emotional distress are common initial reactions to a diagnosis of genital herpes. A painful first episode can lead to a severe grief reaction for loss of health and personal image. Initial shock and emotional numbing, a sense of isolation and loneliness, anger directed at the individual thought to be the source of the infection, fear about the long-term consequences of the condition on sexuality and feelings of contamination are all linked to the stages of the grief process patients may go through.

Recurrent genital herpes can have a particularly pervasive negative effect on the individual concerned. Some patients become more deeply depressed with each recurrence and there is a tendency for herpes to be regarded as a personal handicap. The patient often feels anger towards friends and relatives for being insensitive and anguish regarding relationships with non-sufferers, who they do not want to infect (Drob, Loemer & Lifschutz, 1985).

Sufferers find it especially distressing that the condition cannot be cured and they may experience a feeling of loss of control over their lives. This in turn can lead to feelings of despair and helplessness. Others describe the disease as a punishment or a sign of personal weakness. Women may have additional fears about fertility, the development of cervical cancer or of passing the virus on to their children (Oates, 1990).

Most people who suffer from recurrent episodes report a profound effect on their sexual functioning, attributable to the disease. Although their libido remains unaltered, many patients experience reduced pleasure from intercourse, because of the fear and anxiety of passing the virus to partners (Drob, Loemer & Lifshutz, 1985). Fear of rejection can cause a loss of sexual confidence, which may lead to difficulty in forming new relationships. This can then affect the patient's capacity for physical warmth as well as intimacy. When the disease occurs in young people who are developing sexually, the condition can have a devastating effect.

Few people who have genital herpes feel confident enough to talk to people from whom they would normally seek support and comfort, for example family, friends, spouse or sexual partner.

Moral issues arise when considering whether or when to inform new or current sexual partners. This is further complicated by problems associated with determining when one is infectious (Oates, 1990) and because of this, some patients feel that celibacy is their only reasonable option and is preferable to being rejected. Other people respond to the disease by limiting sexual intimacy to those from outside their social circle, so that friends do not find out about their condition, or by choosing casual sexual partners in whom they have little interest, so that they are not disappointed later (Drob, Loemer & Lifshutz, 1985).

Genital herpes and pregnancy

In some areas of the USA, neonatal HSV infection complicates 0.02–0.07% of live births, but in the UK it appears to be rare. The reason for this difference is not known (Cleator & Klapper, 1994).

Women who have a first episode of genital herpes during the first trimester may have an increased risk of spontaneous abortion or delivering babies of low birth weight, which is thought to be due to the viraemia that occurs at the time of infection (Whitley et al., 1980). If the pregnancy continues, it is likely that these women will develop sufficient HSV neutralising antibodies (which are usually considered to be at a maximum level 12 weeks after acquisition of the infection) to give the neonate some degree of protection via placental transfer during delivery. Women who have first episodes during the first trimester and early second trimester should be monitored throughout the remainder of the pregnancy to see if recurrences occur. The risk of a recurrence occurring during the third trimester or at term has been estimated to be over 50% (Woolley et al., 1988).

Pregnant women who have a history of genital herpes prior to conception, as well as those having first episodes during the first and early second trimester, should be examined early in labour (Corey, 1990). Whenever possible, samples should be taken from lesions for viral studies and if a suspicious lesion is seen and/or genital herpes is suspected, then a caesarean section may be considered (Woolley et al., 1988).

If first episode genital herpes occurs late in the third trimester, a caesarean section is strongly recommended, as there is a higher risk of neonatal infection (Oates, 1990). The nearer the time of delivery that the infection occurs, the greater the risk of neonatal infection, as the mother will produce only a low level of antibodies to be passed on to the baby. When born to a mother with recurrent episodes of HSV, the risk to the neonate has been estimated to be between 3% and 5% and may be up to 30–40% (Overall et al., 1984). However, it has now been shown that the majority of mothers of neonates infected with HSV had no previous history of genital herpes (Whitley et al., 1980).

Antiviral therapies

A number of antiviral agents have been used to treat genital herpes. Idoxuridine, as a 5% solution in dimethyl sulphoxide, applied topically and vidarabine (adenosine arabinoside) were commonly used in the pre-aciclovir era but their efficacy was limited by their side effects (Oates, 1990). Topical foscarnet may be used to treat HSV strains resistant to aciclovir (Corey, 1990).

Aciclovir was first synthesised in 1974 and was a major step forward in herpes research, as it is capable of specifically inhibiting viral DNA replication while leaving the host DNA functioning normally. It has a proven safety record because of its selectivity. Aciclovir is drawn to enter HSV-infected cells, where it is converted into aciclovir monophosphate, aciclovir diphosphate and finally to aciclovir triphosphate (Cleator & Klapper, 1994). Aciclovir triphosphate is incorporated into the growing viral DNA strand, which halts further chain elongation and hence viral replication is halted.

Initially, oral aciclovir was only recommended for patients with first episodes and at a dose of 200 mg five times daily for 5 days. Kinghorn et al. (1983) found that topical aciclovir 5% cream was an effective treatment for first episode and recurrent genital herpes. However, as cream is difficult to keep applied to the genital area and as it was found to be less effective than oral therapy, it has now been superseded by patient-initiated episodic courses of oral aciclovir, in similar doses to those used for first episodes. There is no advantage in combining oral and topical therapy in the treatment of first episodes (Kinghorn et al., 1986).

Initial assessment prior to the commencement of continuous suppressive therapy frequently includes a full blood count, liver function tests and renal function tests. However, haematological abnormalities, hepatotoxicity and nephrotoxicity have not been problems in patients with frequently recurring genital herpes who have received continuous therapy for up to 2 years (Mertz et al., 1988). Although aciclovir has not been found to have teratogenic properties, female patients are advised to use a reliable method of contraception while taking continuous therapy. However, conceiving while taking aciclovir therapy is not an indication for terminating the pregnancy.

The optimal starting dose for suppression is 200 mg four times daily, but as compliance is poor, 400 mg twice daily is often prescribed. For patients who remain free from recurrences, it may be possible to reduce the aciclovir to a lower daily dose while still achieving viral suppression (Mindel et al., 1988). The use of frequent daily doses is superior to the use of a high single daily dose, though compliance is a problem.

Some people may continue to experience recurrences while on suppressive doses of aciclovir and for these people the dose can be doubled to 800 mg twice daily (Mindel et al., 1988). However, because systemic absorption is rate-limited, doubling the dose does not result in twice the plasma level and breakthrough recurrences may still occur despite the higher dose. Recurrences that occur when the patient is on this increased dose may indicate malabsorption of the drug, and plasma aciclovir levels may be of value in determining whether this is the case. After stopping continuous therapy patients should be kept under observation and asked to record the subsequent pattern of recurrences.

New generation antivirals

Two new antiviral agents active against herpes viruses, which are reported to have low toxicity, are now licensed for use in treating genital herpes.

Valaciclovir (Valtrex), the 1-valyl ester of aciclovir, is rapidly and almost completely (99%) converted to aciclovir by liver enzymes

(Woolley, 1995). He also notes that when given orally, it results in a three to four times greater plasma level of aciclovir when compared with orally administered aciclovir and as it is an ester of aciclovir, the only by-product of the conversion of valaciclovir to aciclovir is the naturally occurring amino acid 1-valine. As valaciclovir is a prodrug of aciclovir, preclinical and clinical safety data suggest there are similar safety profiles for the two agents.

Famciclovir (Famvir) is a prodrug of penciclovir. It has a similar spectrum of activity to aciclovir and delivers a high concentration of penciclovir to HSV-infected cells (SmithKline Beecham, 1995). Phosphorylation of penciclovir to the triphosphate form is similar to aciclovir and is highly dependent on the thymidine kinase produced by HSV. In herpes-infected cells, penciclovir triphosphate remains in a high concentration despite a lower plasma concentration. SmithKline Beecham (1995) state that oral famciclovir is rapidly absorbed and the active agent, penciclovir, is eliminated rapidly and almost completely by the kidneys.

Molluscum contagiosum

Transmission and presentation

Molluscum contagiosum is a benign papular condition of the skin and mucous membranes characterised by umbilicated papules that tend to be on the face, trunk and extremities in children and in the genital area in adults (Neff, 1990). It appears to be transmitted by direct contact with skin of infected individuals and/or fomites (Coleman, 1990), and non-sexual transmission has also been reported in association with contact sports, swimming and the use of gymnastic equipment and towels (Robertson, McMillan & Young, 1989).

In adults, molluscum contagiosum commonly affects the thigh, lower abdomen and genital areas (Adler, 1990). In the UK, there is a peak incidence at age 24 due to sexual transmission (Coleman, 1990), which is similar to the peak incidence of other STDs. There is also a peak incidence in the UK between the ages of 10 and 15 years, which is probably due to transmission by fomites (Coleman, 1990).

Molluscum contagiosum is a pox virus which produces characteristic inclusion bodies. The virus itself is compact and brick-shaped with a dumb-bell-shaped nucleoid. The nucleoid is surrounded by the inner and outer membranes of the virus particle with the two lateral bodies lying between the inner and outer membrane (Brown, Nalley & Kraus, 1981).

Clinical features

Researchers feel that the incubation period varies, with ranges from 14–50 days (Coleman, 1990) to 2–12 weeks (Adler, 1990). Lesions begin as pinpoint papules that enlarge to form smooth, firm, flesh-coloured papules with a characteristic central umbilication from which caseous material can be expressed (Robertson, McMillan & Young, 1989). Coleman (1990) suggests that the papules may enlarge to 5–10 mm over 6 to 12 weeks, but occasionally the 'giant molluscum' up to 1.5 cm in size, is seen in immunosuppressed patients such as those with HIV/AIDS .

Most people do not have symptoms unless there is a secondary infection (Wilkin, 1977). Some experience itching or tenderness over the lesions, though where lesions appear in crops, auto–inoculation may be a factor (Schofield, 1979).

In the immunocompetent, the number of individual lesions varies from one to 20 (Brown, Nalley & Kraus, 1981) and rarely exceeds 100. The number and distribution of lesions may increase if there is an underlying skin disorder, for example atopic eczema or contact dermatitis; if steroid creams have recently been used; or if there is a coexistent immunosuppressive disorder caused by either drugs or disease (Brown, Nalley & Kraus, 1981; Neff, 1990).

Bacterial superinfection has been shown to complicate the course of molluscum contagiosum infection, leading to symptoms that cause the patient to seek medical attention. Kipping (1971) found that up to 10% of patients seen consecutively developed molluscum dermatitis between 1 and 15 months after the initial onset of viral lesions. He found an inflammatory response, but not all the papules were involved and biopsy showed molluscum bodies with lymphocytes and small round cells, forming an inflammatory infiltrate in the dermis.

Wilkin (1977) found no cases of materno–fetal transmission, though he found evidence to suggest an increase in the number of lesions during pregnancy, which was difficult to evaluate fully due to the small number of patients, but he concluded that this was likely to be due to changes in the immune status of the pregnant woman. He also found that lesions had not developed in the infants of women in whom follow-up was possible. Mandel and Lewis (1970) reported lesions on a neonate of 1 week old. However, there was no history of infectious disease and no lesions of molluscum contagiosum on the parents or on the child at birth. Although the parents were apparently free of the condition, the authors concluded that the possibility of vaginal transmission could not be ruled out by current diagnostic methods at the time.

Katzman et al. (1987) described the clinical and immunological details of two cases of molluscum contagiosum occurring in patients with acquired immune deficiency syndrome (AIDS) and concluded that the virus may act as an opportunistic pathogen in such patients. They observed that the distribution of lesions was similar to that found in childhood molluscum contagiosum, in contrast to the pattern of genital lesions normally found in adults described by Brown, Nalley and Kraus (1981).

Pathogenesis

Robertson, McMillan and Young (1989) note that molluscum lesions appear as a mass of hyperplastic and hypertrophied epidermis that extends down into the dermis, though it does not breach the basement membrane, while above the surface the papule can be seen. Coleman (1990) notes that molluscum contagiosum replicates in the cytoplasm of the inclusion bodies, which migrate in the infected cells through the dermal layer, leading to the core of a lesion consisting of inclusion bodies, keratin and degenerating epidermal cells (Robertson, McMillan & Young, 1989).

A major problem of investigating pathogenesis of molluscum contagiosum is that it does not grow at all well on tissue culture, it has not been transmitted to laboratory animals and it will not grow in eggs (Coleman, 1990).

Diagnosis

The diagnosis of molluscum contagiosum is usually made clinically (Coleman, 1990) though it can be made histologically by observing molluscum bodies in biopsy specimens (Katzman et al., 1987). Other diagnostic procedures include the detection of molluscum contagiosum antigen using fluorescent antibody tests and visualisation of virus particles by electron microscopy or by Giemsa staining (Brown, Nalley & Kraus, 1981; Robertson, McMillan & Young, 1989).

Treatment

Individual lesions of molluscum contagiosum usually resolve spontaneously within 6–9 months but occasionally they may take as long as 3–4 years (Coleman, 1990).

Treatment is usually aimed at eradicating the lesions by some form of mechanical destruction, though spontaneous resolution, frequent recurrences and the benign nature of the condition must be weighed against the side effects of treatment, namely local pain and potential for tissue scarring (Brown, Nalley & Kraus, 1981).

Robertson, McMillan and Young (1989) note that it is not necessary to completely remove the lesion but just to open the core to allow resolution to occur. No form of destructive therapy has been shown to be superior to any other. Brown, Nalley and Kraus (1981) note that freezing, chemicals or electric current may be used to damage the papule, leading to resolution, and various methods have been used. The simplest method consists of expression of the core of the lesion, either by direct pressure or curettage, followed by cauterisation of the base. Alternatively, cryotherapy can be used, either by the application of a cotton wool-tipped swab that has been soaked in liquid nitrogen or by using a cryotherapy probe cooled by nitrous oxide. For small lesions, topical preparations can be used, for example phenol or iodine (Coleman, 1990), though trichloroacetic acid is used in some clinics.

Bacterial superinfection should be treated with systemic antibiotics and as with all STDs, screening for other genital infections should be performed and sexual contacts may be advised to attend. Coleman (1990) notes that the patient should be seen 2–3 weeks after the initial treatment, as new lesions may have appeared or lesions may have been missed.

Useful address

Herpes Viruses Association (Sphere), 41 North Road, London N7 9PD. Tel: 0171 607 9661 (office); 0171 609 9061 (helpline).

References

Adler MW (1990) ABC of Sexually Transmitted Diseases. London: British Medical Association.

Ashley RL, Militoni J, Lee F, Nahmias A, Corey L (1988) Comparison of Western Blot (Immunoblot) and Glycoprotein G-specific Immunodot enzyme assay for detecting antibodies to *Herpes simplex* virus types 1 and 2 in human sera. Journal of Clinical Microbiology 26(4): 662–7.

Brown ST, Nalley JF, Kraus SJ (1981) Molluscum contagiosum. Sexually Transmitted Diseases 8(3): 227–34.

Cleater GM, Klapper PE (1994) *Herpes simplex*. In Zuckerman AJ, Banatrala JE, Pattison JR (Eds), Principles and Practice of Clinical Urology 3rd edn. Chichester: John Wiley & Sons

Coleman JC (1990) Cytomegalovirus, infectious mononucleosis and molluscum contagiosum. In Csonka GW, Oates JK (Eds), Sexually Transmitted Diseases – A Textbook of Genitourinary Medicine. London: Baillière Tindall.

Conant MA, Spicer DW, Smith CD (1984) *Herpes simplex* virus transmission: condom studies. Sexually Transmitted Diseases 11(2): 94–5.

Corey L (1990) Genital herpes. In Holmes KK, Mårdh P-A, Sparling PF, Wiesner PJ (Eds), Sexually Transmitted Diseases, 2nd edn. New York: McGraw-Hill.

Cowan FM, Johnson AM, Ashley R, Corey L, Mindel A (1994) Antibody to *Herpes simplex* virus type 2 as serological marker of sexual lifestyle in populations. British Medical Journal 309: 1325–9.

DOH (1995) Sexually Transmitted Diseases, England 1994. Department of Health Statistical Bulletin. London: HMSO.

Drob S, Loemer M, Lifshutz H (1985) Genital herpes: the psychological consequences. British Journal of Medical Psychology 58: 307–15.

Katzman M, Carey JT, Elmets CA, Jacobs GH, Lederman MM (1987) Molluscum contagiosum and the acquired immunodeficiency syndrome: clinical and immunological details of two cases. British Journal of Dermatology 116: 131–8.

Kinghorn GR, Turner EB, Barton IG, Potter CW, Burke CA, Fiddian AP (1983) Efficacy of topical acyclovir cream in first and recurrent episodes of genital herpes. Antiviral Research 3: 291–301.

Kinghorn GR, Abeywickreme I, Jeavons M, Barton I, Potter CW, Jones D, Hickmott E (1986) Efficacy of combined treatment with oral and topical acyclovir in first episode genital herpes. Genitourinary Medicine 62(1): 186–8.

Kipping HF (1971) Molluscum dermatitis. Archive of Dermatology 103: 106–7.

Koutsky LA, Stevens CE, Holmes KK, Ashley RL, Kiviat NB, Critchlow CW, Corey L (1992) Underdiagnosis of genital herpes by current clinical and viral-isolation procedures. New England Journal of Medicine 326(23): 1533–9.

Lafferty WE, Krofft S, Remington M, Giddings R, Winter C, Cent A, Corey L (1987) Diagnosis of *Herpes simplex* virus by direct immunofluorescence and viral isolation from samples of external genital lesions in a high-prevalence population. Journal of Clinical Microbiology 25(2): 323–6.

Mandel MJ, Lewis RJ (1970) Molluscum contagiosum of the newborn. British Journal of Dermatology 84: 370–2.

Mertz GJ, Eron L, Kaufman R, Goldberg L, Raab B, Conant M, Mills J, Kurtz T, Davis LG (1988) Prolonged continuous versus intermittent oral acyclovir treatment in normal adults with frequently recurring genital *Herpes simplex* virus infection. American Journal of Medicine 85(supplement 2A): 14–19.

Mindel A, Faherty A, Carney O, Patou G, Freris M, Williams P (1988) Dosage and safety of long-term suppressive acyclovir therapy for recurrent genital herpes. Lancet April 23: 926–8.

Neff JM (1990) Parapoxviruses and molluscum contagiosum and tanapox virses. In Mandell GL, Douglas RG, Bennett JE (Eds), Principles and Practice of Infectious Diseases, 3rd edn. New York: Churchill Livingstone.

Oates JK (1990) Anogenital herpes. In Csonka GW, Oates JK (Eds), Sexually Transmitted Diseases – A Textbook of Genitourinary Medicine. London: Baillière Tindall.

Overall JC, Whitley RJ, Yeager AS, McCracken GH, Nelson JD (1984) Prophylactic or anticipatory antiviral therapy for newborns exposed to *Herpes simplex* infection. Pediatric Infectious Disease 3(3): 193–5.

Rattray MC, Corey L, Reeves WC, Vontver LA, Holmes KK (1978) Recurrent genital herpes among women: symptomatic v. asymptomatic viral shedding. British Journal of Venereal Diseases 54: 262–5.

Robertson DHH, McMillan A, Young H (1989) Clinical Practice in Sexually Transmissible Diseases, 2nd edn. Edinburgh: Churchill Livingstone.

Schofield CBS (1979) Sexually Transmitted Diseases, 3rd edn. Edinburgh: Churchill Livingstone.

Shelley WB (1967) *Herpes simplex* virus as a cause of erythema multiforme. JAMA 201(3): 153–6.

SmithKline Beecham (1995) Famvir. In ABPI Datasheet Compendium. London: Datapharm Publications.

Whitley RJ, Nahmias AJ, Visintine AM, Fleming CL, Alford CA (1980) The natural history of *Herpes simplex* virus infection of mother and newborn. Pediatrics 66(4): 489–94.

Wilkin JK (1977) Molluscum contagiosum venereum in a women's outpatient clinic: a venereally transmitted disease. American Journal of Obstetrics and Gynecology 128(5): 531–5.

Woolley PD (1991) Value of examining the sexual partners of women suffering from initial genital herpes. International Journal of STD & AIDS 2: 365–6.

Woolley PD (1995) Recent advances in antiviral therapy. British Journal of Sexual Medicine 22(4): 14–15.

Woolley PD, Bowman CA, Hicks DA, Kinghorn GR (1988) Virological screening for *Herpes simplex* virus during pregnancy. British Medical Journal 296: 1642–3.

Woolley PD, Chandiok S (undated) Survey of the management of genital herpes in general practice. (Unpublished.)

Woolley PD, Kudesia G (1990) Incidence of *Herpes simplex* virus type-1 and type-2 from patients with primary (first-attack) genital herpes in Sheffield. International Journal of STD & AIDS 1: 184–6.

Chapter 10
HIV and AIDS

Jean Hale and Alison Sutton

Introduction

There are many books on the nursing and medical care of people infected with the human immunodeficiency virus (HIV) and those who have acquired immune deficiency syndrome (AIDS). Therefore, this chapter will concentrate on certain aspects of nursing care relevant to nurses in genito-urinary medicine (GUM) clinics and mention other aspects only briefly. In areas where there are a large number of HIV-positive patients there is often a separate HIV clinic, however, many GUM clinic nurses are providing all the care in areas where prevalence is low.

History and prevalence

The early story of the recognition of HIV and AIDS is well known. In 1981, a group of young homosexual men in the USA were found to have pneumonia caused by *Pneumocystis carinii*, while another group of homosexual men were diagnosed with Kaposi's sarcoma. As both these conditions were virtually unknown in young, healthy, immunocompetent people, investigations were made and it was discovered that all the men were immunodeficient (Pratt, 1995). By September 1982 the disease had become known as AIDS and had also been recognised in the UK (Illman, 1993).

The identification of the virus that causes AIDS was made in 1983 and 1984 by two groups of workers, who called their discoveries lymphadenopathy associated virus (LAV) and human lymphotrophic virus type III (HLTV III). Once it was recognised that these were very similar, the designation human immunodeficiency virus (HIV)

was made (Loveday, 1996). Two strains of HIV have now been identified, HIV-1, which is the predominant strain worldwide, particularly in the USA and Europe, and HIV-2, which is generally found
only in parts of Africa.

When reporting of HIV and AIDS was first started in the UK, it
appeared to be confined to homosexual men, however, Murray and
Johnson (1996) believe that an estimated 65% of HIV infection
worldwide up to 1992 is thought to have been from heterosexual
transmission, with a projection of 80–90% of the transmission by the
year 2000. They note that the pattern of the HIV epidemic is very
different in different parts of the world, with 50–75% of the cases of
AIDS being reported in homosexual or bisexual men in the USA
and the UK and injecting drug users making up 60% of the cases in
southern Europe; while in Asia and Africa, the epidemic is mainly
heterosexual, though it seems to have started in female sex workers
and drug users.

The World Health Organization (WHO) collates information
about HIV infection and AIDS from all over the world, though it is
known that the accuracy of reporting varies greatly. In the developed world, reporting is fairly accurate. However, there is believed
to be serious under-reporting in other parts of the world, particularly
Africa, due to limited diagnostic and reporting procedures. WHO
(1995) has reported over a million cases of AIDS and estimated that
there would be more than 4.5 million cases of AIDS by mid-1995.
In addition, it estimates that 18–19 million adults and more than 1.5
million children were infected with HIV between the 1970s and
mid-1995. It is estimated that 30–40 million adults and children will
be infected with HIV worldwide by the year 2000, with 90% found
in developing countries (Murray & Johnson, 1996).

In the UK, surveillance is coordinated by the Communicable
Disease Surveillance Centre (CDSC), who report that from 1982,
when reporting began, to February 1996, there have been 12 201
cases of AIDS in the UK (11 031 men and 1 170 women), 70% of
whom have died. The number of people reported as infected with
HIV-1 up to the end of 1995 was 25 689 and there was a 13%
increase in new infections in 1995 against 1994 figures (CDSC,
1996).

Transmission and risk

The Royal College of Nursing HIV Nursing Society (RCN) (1994)
note that HIV is not contagious but infectious and that social

interaction, close personal contact, insects, etc. have not been shown to cause spread of HIV infection. The routes of transmission of HIV infection have been categorised by Pratt (1995) as follows:

- sexual transmission;
- vertical transmission;
- drug use;
- iatrogenic transmission.

HIV has been found in semen and cervical secretions, as well as tears, saliva, urine, breast milk, lymphocytes in the peripheral blood, cerebrospinal fluid and cell-free plasma, and sexual transmission can be through unprotected anal or vaginal intercourse, in both homosexuals and heterosexuals (Murray & Johnson, 1996). In the West, the majority of infections seen initially were in gay or bisexual men, but Singh and Cusack (1994) note that worldwide HIV is spread heterosexually seven times more than homosexually and that about 75% of infections worldwide are from sexual transmission, with women making up 30% and the ratio of female to male rising quickly.

Vertical transmission is from mother to child and the RCN (1994) note that it may happen trans-placentally *in utero*, during the process of labour and birth or during the neonatal period, as well as through breast milk, particularly if the mother is infected during the time she is breastfeeding.

Iatrogenic transmission is from blood and blood products such as Factor VIII, which is used to treat haemophilia, and from organ transplants and artificial insemination with donated semen (Pratt, 1995).

It is now thought that various co-factors affect the risk of being infected with HIV at any particular episode of exposure. Pratt (1995) notes that the type of sexual activity affects the risk, with male to female by vaginal or anal intercourse and active male to passive male by anal intercourse, or occasionally oral sex fellatio, being more likely to cause transmission than female to male or passive male to active male intercourse. He suggests that other factors include the viral load or amount of virus a person is exposed to; the stage in the disease of the HIV-positive person – early in the infection and then when symptoms occur appear to be the times when there is highest risk of transmission; the presence of other sexually transmitted diseases (STDs), particularly where there is ulceration; bleeding during intercourse; and the number of sexual partners – the more partners one has, the higher the risk of being infected with HIV.

As discussed earlier, it is important to recognise that the pattern of HIV infection varies from country to country.

Pathogenesis and progression

HIV is a retrovirus. Structurally, it has an outer envelope and an inner capsid, and it carries its genetic message as RNA. A reverse transcriptase enzyme allows the virus to turn RNA into DNA when it enters the host cell (Loveday, 1996).

Singh (1994) notes that HIV targets particular lymphocytes within the immune system, known as CD4 cells or T-helper cells. As these lymphocytes are activated in response to any infection or antigenic compounds, such as Factor VIII, over time more and more cells are infected and the immune response decreases, leaving the body open to infection (Pratt, 1995).

It is believed that HIV may have originated from a similar disease in monkeys in Africa, which made a species leap to humans, probably hundreds of years ago and gradually the infection has spread to become an epidemic and then a pandemic infection (Pratt, 1995). Pratt (1995) goes on to suggest that the disease is now seen as a progression with various phases and Singh (1994) notes that it is believed that once a person is infected with HIV they will eventually develop symptoms, though they may not do so for many years. Murray and Johnson (1996) suggest that studies of haemophiliacs and gay men in the developed world show that 50% of people with HIV will develop AIDS after 10 years and 60% after 13–14 years, though it is known that this is very variable, with some patients developing symptomatic infection either much sooner or much later.

Pratt (1995) has described six stages in HIV disease.

Phase A – acute HIV infection

Two to six weeks after being infected with HIV, some people have a flu/glandular fever-like illness, referred to as seroconversion illness, which is the result of the body's immune response to being infected. Patients may have a fever, rash, headache, malaise, etc.

Phase B – antibody positive phase

Phase B-1 asymptomatic HIV infection. Many patients appear to be asymptomatic though changes can be seen in their blood and immune system. This phase has been referred to as a latent phase in the past, but work by Ho et al. (1995) and Wei et al. (1995) has shown that during this phase, there is very rapid continuous replication of HIV, which causes a rapid turnover of CD4 cells.

Phase B-2 persistent generalised lymphadenopathy (PGL). Some patients have lymph node enlargement for many years, without further clinical signs.

Phase C – early symptomatic disease

This phase used to be referred to as AIDS-related complex (ARC), however, this is now considered outdated (Singh, 1994). Patients in this phase of HIV disease may have various minor infections which may lead them to be chronically ill. Skin conditions, hairy leucoplakia, herpes, malnutrition and oral candidiasis are common.

Phase D – late symptomatic disease (AIDS)

Ho et al. (1995) believe that the high level of virus replication and destruction of CD4 lymphocytes lead to the development of AIDS in the continuum of the disease. The list of AIDS defining conditions as described by the Centers for Disease Control (CDC) is shown in Table 10.1.

Phases E – remission; and F – terminal illness

In between bouts of opportunistic infection or a condition found in AIDS, the patient may improve and be in a stage of remission, before moving eventually to a terminal phase.

HIV antibody testing

In the UK, an antibody test has been available since 1985 and most Western countries routinely offer HIV antibody testing, though it is not so widely available in developing countries (McCreaner, 1989).

It is impossible to look for the virus itself and therefore it is antibodies produced in reaction to infection which are tested for, though Mortimer (1993) notes that occasionally cross-reactions occur that may lead to false-positive results. He goes on to discuss that for this reason, all positive results should be confirmed by a different form of test and a second sample of blood should be taken and tested as further confirmation, preferably by a different laboratory.

Table 10.1: AIDS defining diagnosis, classified by CDC (RCN, 1994)

Indicator disease

Adults
Candidiasis of trachea, bronchi, oesophagus
Coccidioidomycosis: disseminated or extrapulmonary
Crytococcosis: extrapulmonary
Crytosporidiosis: diarrhoea over 1 month
Cytomegalovirus retinitis
Cytomegalovirus disease
HIV encephalopathy
Herpes simplex virus (HSV): bronchitis, pneumonitis, oesophagitis after age 1 month
Histoplasmosis
Isosporiasis: diarrhoea over 1 month
Mycobacterial disease: including extrapulmonary tuberculosis and disseminated
Mycobacterial infection, atypical
Pneumocystis carinii pneumonia
Progressive multifocal leucoencephalopathy
Toxoplasmosis: cerebral
Salmonella (non-typhoid) septicaemia: recurrent
Wasting syndrome due to HIV fever
Recurrent pneumonia in a 12-month period

AIDS indicator neoplasms
Kaposi's sarcoma
Primary central nervous system lymphoma, non-Hodgkin's lymphoma
Cervical carcinoma: invasive

Children
Bacterial infections: multiple or recurrent, in child aged up to 12
Lymphoid interstitial pneumonia: in child aged up to 12

The RCN (1994) note that the three main types of test used are enzyme-linked immunosorbent assays (ELISA), radio-immunoassays (RIA) and Western Blot tests. ELISA tests are also known as enzyme immunoassays (EIA) and they are the commonest HIV antibody test in use (Pratt, 1995). Mortimer (1993) notes that ELISA tests are generally very sensitive.

IgG (or gammaglobulin) antibodies are made by the body in response to the glycoprotein (gp41) found on the outer coating of HIV. Because these antibodies are long-lasting, they are used as a marker and ELISA tests look for them along with the protein (p24) found in the core of the virus (Pratt, 1995).

RIA tests or immunofluorescent assay (IFA) are used more for research than testing, as they take longer and are technically more difficult to carry out than ELISA tests. Therefore the Western Blot test is generally used to confirm the diagnosis (Pratt, 1995), though Mortimer (1993) believes that many laboratories in the UK tend to use a machine-read assay for confirmation, rather than Western Blotting.

Antigen tests are also available, though not usually used for diagnosis but for determining prognosis, as antigens reappear in symptomatic infection (Pratt, 1995). He also notes that a recent development is the rapid method test, which may be done on urine or saliva samples and which does not need laboratory equipment. However, there are many ethical considerations to such tests, as people could do a test at home for themselves without counselling and support.

Counselling for HIV antibody testing

The Health of the Nation document (DOH, 1993) states that a person must give explicit informed consent to have named testing for HIV and that pre-test discussion or counselling should therefore be given before testing is undertaken and post-test counselling given following the result. Pratt (1995) notes that informed consent means that the person knows why a test is being done and that time and space are needed for the patient to understand the information being given.

Many other workers, such as voluntary support groups or women's health group workers, may have discussions or counselling with people without carrying out testing (DOH, 1993) and many patients prefer to prepare for testing in this way. Some workers feel that pre-test counselling for HIV antibody testing is often an information-giving and preparation exercise as much as counselling.

People may have HIV antibody testing for various reasons. The RCN (1994) suggests that the main reason is that individuals believe that they may have put themselves at risk of being infected with HIV. Sometimes a patient may be advised to have an HIV antibody test because of their clinical condition or because a health care worker feels the patient may have been exposed to HIV. Often the patient may be due to have an invasive procedure that may be perceived as causing extra hazards to staff. Also, many haemophiliacs have been infected with HIV from contaminated Factor VIII and they may request an HIV antibody test.

Pratt (1995) notes the following six points as benefits of having a test, if a person believes they may have been exposed to HIV because of their past lifestyle:

1.   Testing allows a person to be given health education and indi-
     vidual counselling and people who have a negative test should
     be reassured and therefore committed to keeping themselves
     safe.

2.   Treatment can be given to slow disease progression, with regu-
     lar monitoring of CD4 cells, if a person is positive.

3.   Prophylaxis for opportunistic infections can be given if a
     person knows their HIV status.

4.   If a person knows they are HIV-positive while asymptomatic,
     they can be vaccinated against infections such as hepatitis B
     and flu.

5.   Women who are HIV-positive are believed to be more at risk
     of cervical dysplasia and therefore need frequent cervical
     cytology. In addition, women may wish to know their status to
     help them make decisions regarding their children.

6.   Lastly, decisions about certain medical procedures and treat-
     ments may be affected by HIV status, for example transplant
     surgery would not be offered to an HIV-positive patient.

However, Pratt (1995) also notes that there are disadvantages of
being tested for an individual person:

1.   Some people may not follow safer sex practices if they have
     had a negative HIV result, as they believe they are not at risk.

2.   People who are HIV-positive may suffer from discrimination
     and prejudice and their status may affect insurance, travel,
     relationships with partners, family, etc. Equally, some people
     who are negative may be treated as having a risky lifestyle,
     regardless of the result.

3.   Some people find it difficult to adjust psychologically to a posi-
     tive result and therefore do not cope well with their disease.

Much has been written on the attitudes needed to undertake a
counselling role, so only a few points will be made in relation to this.
Bor, Miller and Goldman (1992) note that the ability to recognise
each patient as an individual with different therapeutic needs, to see
each patient as unique, to approach patients with openness and to
listen are all important aspects of skilful couselling. Empathetic
counselling, which allows the patient to dictate the pace while listening and trying to understand what the patient thinks and feels about
a problem is another important component of counselling, as is
recognising that everyone makes judgments and has preconceived

ideas but what matters is the ability to put these to one side and care for the patient (Bor, Miller & Goldman, 1992). Equally, if a counsellor has a problem putting aside their own judgments with a particular patient, then referral to another worker would be appropriate. Pratt (1995) points out that hospitals should ensure that effective pre- and post-test counselling is carried out by trained staff, with time and space to carry out the counselling.

Pre-test counselling

McCreaner (1989) notes that as pre-test counselling involves detailed discussion of intimate and normally private parts of a person's life, trust between the patient and counsellor is paramount. The RCN (1994) suggest that the following points need to be covered in pre-test counselling:

- why the person wants a test and what the result will mean to that person;
- the issue of confidentiality and who knows the result;
- problems of insurance, isolation, pregnancy and travel;
- what support a person is likely to have and if they are ready for a positive result if it occurs.

Bor, Miller and Goldman (1992) suggest that the patient needs to be made aware of the confidentiality in counselling for HIV testing at the start of the session and *The Health of the Nation* document (DOH, 1993) also stresses the confidential nature of counselling and that information, specimen labelling, etc., must be adhered to, as required by the NHS Venereal Disease Regulations 1974.

To explore why a person wants to have a test, it is necessary to find out what the person knows about transmission and risk of HIV infection and what he or she believes to be the risk (Bor, Miller & Goldman, 1992). McCreaner (1989) suggests that the counsellor should be aware of not jumping to conclusions about risk factors, as these may change over time and although people may be considered to be at 'low risk', they are very rarely at 'no risk'. Bor, Miller and Goldman (1992) note that it is important to clarify exactly what is meant by sex, whether it is kissing, cuddling, vaginal, oral or anal intercourse, as it will be different for each individual and the risk associated with various activities differs. The patient may need to be advised about the ways HIV can be transmitted.

When looking at the test itself and the result, many patients are still under the misconception that the HIV test is an AIDS test and the difference between being infected with HIV and having AIDS has to be explained clearly (McCreaner, 1989). An important factor at this stage is understanding of the window period, the 6–12 week period that is known to occur between infection and antibody production and this is particularly important when the result is negative (Bor, Miller & Goldman, 1992). Pratt (1995) notes that a patient may have a negative test, but if they are in the window period, they may be not only infected but infectious to sexual contacts. Also, some people may take up to 6 months for seroconversion and very rarely, a person may not show antibodies on testing, even though they have been infected with HIV. *The Health of the Nation* document (DOH, 1993) states that results must be given in person and with the shortest wait possible, to reduce anxiety.

Most people who come for HIV testing believe they are negative, therefore they have considered the implications of a negative result but not what a positive result would mean (McCreaner, 1989). The patient needs to think through the implications of having a test and a positive result and it is important to prepare the patient for a positive result, whatever the risk factors (Bor, Miller & Goldman, 1992). The problems of isolation and who to tell if the result is positive, as well as the support that is likely from partners, family and friends, are issues that the patient should address. Bor, Miller and Goldman (1992) note that patients should know that support will be available from HIV workers, such as in a GUM department, during office hours, and that helplines, both local and national, are available at other times. They also suggest that some patients do not think they would be likely to tell their GP, because of concern about obtaining continuing care. However, GPs may see a patient for HIV-related symptoms such as coughs and colds and do need to know the diagnosis.

McCreaner (1989) points out that although the law may protect people from losing their job due to discrimination, a patient may not wish to declare that they are HIV-positive and equally, issues of insurance, mortgage policies, travel visas and so on are also very important to discuss. Bor, Miller and Goldman (1992) believe that a psychological assessment should be made, to ensure that even if the patient is anxious or agitated, which are natural reactions in such circumstances, they are making an informed choice to have a test. Pratt (1995) states that only the patient can make the decision to have a test and that he or she may require more time and space to consider the information and feelings that have come from the counselling session, before having a test.

When ending a pre-test counselling session, the counsellor should allow the patient to ask any questions they want and then make sure the patient knows when the result will be available and that they must attend in person (Bor, Miller & Goldman, 1992).

Post-test counselling

It is important to remember that there is no easy way to give a positive result and that it is best given as soon as possible (Bor, Miller & Goldman, 1992). This post-test session may be the only time one sees the patient, so a lot of information needs to be given. However, Firn and Norman (1995a) identified in their study that receiving a positive diagnosis is one of the times of greatest emotional and psychological impact and no matter how well prepared a patient is, they will almost always be shocked by a positive result and may not be able to take in information that is given or even remember what was said in the pre-test counselling (Bor, Miller & Goldman, 1992). Green (1989) points out that people's reactions can vary greatly and what is important is to listen to the patient and encourage him or her to say what they want about how they feel. The patient needs to understand the implications of a positive result, and to be given hope but also truthful reassurance (Bor, Miller & Goldman, 1992).

Many patients being given a positive diagnosis will worry that they have got AIDS and it is important to reiterate the modes of transmission at this stage, including the fact that social contact, with family, children, neighbours and so on, will not transmit HIV infection (Green, 1989).

It is important to encourage patients to minimise the risk of transmission, which may mean altering behaviour and lifestyle, particularly sexual activity, and safer sex should be discussed in some detail, after finding out exactly what sexual activities the patient has had in the past (Green, 1989). The RCN (1994) points out that the greatest risk is from penetrative vaginal or anal intercourse and that oral sex is much safer, though if there are cuts or sores in the mouth or a woman is menstruating, then the risk of transmission is higher. They suggest that many activities can make sex fun and are very safe, including kissing and licking the body, using sex toys, provided they are not shared, and mutual masturbation; hugging, caressing, touching and massage; tickling, nibbling, lovebites, using mirrors, pictures, fantasies, talking sex; and above all using one's imagination.

Another major element of post-test counselling when giving a positive result is to reassure the patient that their reactions of shock, grief, tears, anger or whatever are normal and that ongoing support is available from the counsellor, the health care team and voluntary agencies (Bor, Miller & Goldman, 1992). The counsellor may need to help the patient to discuss who to tell and how, in relation to partner, parents, friends, etc., which is not a simple matter, as the attitudes and reactions of others are virtually impossible to judge (Green, 1989).

Bor, Miller and Goldman (1992) suggest it is important to discuss medical care, when the patient is ready, as knowledge that monitoring tests are done and treatments can be given to reduce infections may give some hope to the patient. Encouraging the patient to keep well by minimising the risk of contracting infections, whether STDs or respiratory infections, as well as eating well, getting exercise and reducing stress are also part of post-test counselling (Green, 1989).

Finally, a follow-up counselling appointment should be offered, before giving the patient written information and advice and support line numbers (Bor, Miller & Goldman, 1992). The need for support and follow-up is the reason why patients should not be told their result on a Friday, as they may be left without access to such support over the weekend (RCN, 1994).

When a patient receives a negative test result but needs a further test because of the window period, this should be discussed and arranged and there should also be a discussion about safer sex to reduce high-risk behaviour (Bor, Miller & Goldman, 1992).

Partner notification

A particular issue when a patient has tested positive for HIV is that of contact tracing or partner notification. The Health of the Nation document (DOH, 1993) notes that partner notification is standard practice for other STDs and often for HIV and it should be encouraged. Also, the clinic staff should undertake this action when requested to do so by a patient. However, Mackereth and Harrison (1995) have highlighted the concerns nurses have about notifying the partners of patients with HIV and Wright (1996) notes that contact tracing, according to WHO, must not be coercive but voluntary and it must be confidential, which can cause great difficulty where someone who is contacted has only had one or two partners.

However, contact tracing is needed to allow sexual partners to access support, counselling and testing if they wish and to be aware of health problems. Mackereth and Harrison (1995) believe a national protocol with regard to contact tracing in HIV should be developed, but only after consultation with user groups, the public and professional bodies.

Anonymous HIV testing

Anonymous testing for HIV has been carried out to obtain prevalence data from patients attending GUM and antenatal clinics and though patients can opt out, their consent is not needed to include them in the programme (RCN, 1994).

Such testing has been of great concern to nurses and doctors, who feel there are serious ethical implications about trust and the role of professionals, as well as practical implications in interpreting the results (Wright, 1996), and in addition, most health care staff are concerned that anonymous testing means patients who are HIV-positive are not able to access care, take control of their lives and maybe most importantly, reduce transmission to their partners and children.

Same-day testing

The Health of the Nation document (DOH, 1993) highlighted that results of HIV tests should ideally be available within 24 hours. As a result, many GUM clinics have developed same-day testing facilities, whereby patients have the test taken in the morning and receive their result later in the afternoon. However, the service is not available on a Friday, as discussed earlier.

Cameron, Wallis and Blakely (1995) note that the advantages of same-day testing outweigh the disadvantages and although anxiety may not be reduced, its duration is certainly shortened. They also note that many patients find it easier to take a single day off work to attend both appointments, rather than having to attend on two separate days.

The role of the GUM nurse working with HIV-positive patients

The RCN (1994) point out that GUM nurses have great knowledge and expertise in the care of patients with HIV and AIDS, though Hicken and Faugier (1996a) believe that as HIV and AIDS care moves more into the mainstream of care, specialist nurses need to develop advocacy skills, not only for people affected by HIV, but also for generic services and staff. They point out that there is a belief among users of HIV/AIDS services that generic services are not as trustworthy as specialist HIV/AIDS or GUM units. However, if staff working in generic services do not get the chance to care for people affected by HIV, they will not gain experience.

Past research has shown the lack of knowledge and prejudice among nurses about HIV and AIDS, which highlights the need for ongoing education and training (Akinsanya & Rouse, 1992). Hicken and Faugier (1996a) suggest that lifestyle, sexuality and discrimination are more important than fear of being infected for nurses, when caring for patients with HIV. Westcott (1994) highlights that nurses caring for patients with HIV and AIDS may themselves be stigmatised.

Firn and Norman (1995b) interviewed patients with HIV and AIDS to find out their views on the role of the nurse in support of them and identified four elements of the caring role of the nurse:

- providing comfort during a crisis;
- not judging patients with AIDS but just accepting them as they are;
- seeing patients as individuals to respond to;
- using touch while caring.

As patients trust nurses in GUM for their professional expertise, it is important that nurses understand not only the infection but the lifestyle and behaviour of their patients. GUM nurses will care for patients with HIV who have been infected in various ways and often there are special needs associated with each group of patients.

Drug users

Faugier and Hicken (1996a) indicate that attitudes to drug users, especially those who inject drugs, lead to problems for patients being given appropriate accessible care. Loss of continuous contact with drug users is very common and can lead to chaotic treatment patterns (Winship, 1995). Also, many nurses believe that harm minimisation condones drug use, rather than seeing it as a way of working that allows the needs of drug users to be accepted, while enabling nurses to work with them to change to a drug-free lifestyle (RCN, 1994). They point out that many drug users do not know about their own health needs and receive little care and that health and social needs of drug users need to be addressed in a holistic, multidisciplinary approach, to achieve a successful relationship when working with drug users. Coyne and Clancy (1996) believe that the following outcomes can be successfully achieved:

- problem drug users can be enabled to use health and social agencies;
- use of street drugs or multiple drug use can be reduced or stopped;
- penetrative sexual intercourse with regular and casual partners using protection and safer sex practices;
- continuing in or gaining a job;
- relations within the family maintained positively;
- somewhere to live that is stable and continuous.

The RCN (1994) also note that harm minimisation includes the availability of clean injecting equipment and prescription of substitute oral drugs.

Gay and bisexual patients

Statistics for 1994 show that 60–67% of the new HIV infections seen in men in the UK, whether asymptomatic or symptomatic, were homosexually acquired (DOH, 1995). Therefore many patients seen in GUM will be gay or bisexual men. While homophobia is still rife within the general public and particularly the media, Cranfield (1996) notes that many GUM clinics and other services are user-friendly, following strategies to reduce non-attendance rates. Platzer (1993) believes that as partners of gay and lesbian patients have been reported as being denied the status of next-of-kin and, therefore, have not been allowed information or to visit freely during terminal or serious illness, nurses must act as advocates for lesbian and gay patients. In the GUM setting, acceptance and understanding of behaviour and lifestyle in gay and bisexual patients is of extreme importance, to allow positive support and couselling to be offered to such patients with HIV, their partners and significant others.

Sex industry workers

Men and women working in the sex industry are generally well-informed about sexual health issues, safer sex and HIV and AIDS. As risk reduction measures for people with HIV working in the sex industry may mean their financial livelihood is threatened, support and understanding of a patient's lifestyle is very important for GUM nurses.

Pratt (1995) notes that female drug users may resort to prostitution to pay for their drug habit, and in the South Pacific area, international sex tourism has helped the very rapid spread of HIV. Work undertaken in London with male sex industry workers shows that although they may have safer sex with clients, they may not be so safe with private partners who may be women, as not all male workers are gay (Rowe, 1994).

Women and children

The care of women and children with HIV and AIDS may pose particular problems and Westcott (1994) suggests that women need accurate non-judgmental advice on particular issues, such as the risk of transmission to children, safer sex and the problems of dealing with death and dying. Women are often economically dependent on men, with lower status and sexual subordination, and in addition, women are biologically more vulnerable due to the large mucosal area of the vagina and the higher concentration of HIV found in semen than in other body fluids (Pratt, 1995). Also, women may find out through being diagnosed HIV-positive that their partner is bisexual.

Friend (1992) reports that in Europe, 10% of people with HIV and AIDS are women, but in Scotland, the figures are 27% of people with HIV and 12% of those with AIDS. She also notes that women are shown to survive a much shorter time with AIDS than men, possibly due to women coming for treatment later than men, being diagnosed as having AIDS much later as doctors are slower to recognise the symptoms and not being as likely as men to be offered new treatments.

Westcott (1994) points out that women with HIV may be affected by various gynaecological conditions, such as severe pelvic inflammatory disease, genital warts, chronic vaginal candida which does not respond to treatment and abnormal cervical cytology, as well as changes in the menstrual cycle such as dysmenorrhoea, irregular cycles and either heavier or scantier loss.

The risk of transmission of HIV perinatally has been reported by Westcott (1994) as being 13–55% in the USA and western Europe. However, Friend (1992) notes research that suggests a 12% transmission rate. Pratt (1995) discusses how some children, though a decreasing number, are infected by blood products.

Paediatric HIV and AIDS is defined as being in children less than 13 years old. By 1992, 1.1 million children worldwide were reported as being infected with HIV and 575 000 had AIDS (Pratt, 1995). Rees (1995) discusses the fact that infected children may have terminal disease at the same time as their parents, creating extreme distress emotionally.

It is important to remember that maternal antibodies transferred *in utero* mean that all children born to HIV-positive mothers will be HIV-positive at birth and standard HIV antibody tests are therefore not diagnostic until after the age of 18 months, which is why antigen tests, viral cultures and other tests are used to diagnose paediatric infection in the early stages (Pratt, 1995).

Another important issue for GUM nurses is the children affected by HIV as a result of their parents' infection. Plant (1995) suggests that children are affected by stress within the family, even if they do not know the diagnosis. She also describes how a memory store or box with things to help them remember their parents and their childhood will help children. Carlisle (1995) reports on various units such as the Mildmay Mission and St Mary's Paediatric HIV team in London, who have set up specialist care for children infected and affected by HIV.

HIV infection in 13–18-year-olds is likely to occur from either injecting drug use or sexual transmission and Pratt (1995) notes ethical dilemmas for professionals, as it is not clear whether adolescents can give consent for toxic or experimental treatment or whether they can refuse permission for their parents to be told their diagnosis.

Heterosexuals

Heterosexuals who are HIV-positive may feel they are stigmatised by the correlation in the public mind of HIV infection with homosexuality or drug use and they should be treated with as much sensitivity as other groups. As heterosexual transmission is projected to increase, so there is likely to be an increase in the numbers of heterosexuals seen in GUM clinics in future.

Haemophiliacs

Murray and Johnson (1996) report that since screening of all blood and blood products began in the UK in 1985, the HIV infection rate in donors is only 0.001% and that most cases of HIV infection in haemophiliacs occurred in the early 1980s.

Prisoners

Where prisons are situated within the locality of a GUM clinic, nurses may be involved in the care of prisoners. Research has highlighted the fact that homosexual activity is fairly high in prisons, but as prisons are a public place in law, giving prisoners condoms is seen as condoning the illegal act of homosexual sex in a public place (Lineham, 1993). This means that HIV and AIDS prevention in prisons is seriously undermined and as confidentiality in prisons is also a major issue, HIV infection is not being fully addressed in this group of people. GUM nurses should be aware of such issues and provide good safer sex education if the occasion arises.

Infection control guidelines

Much has been written on infection control and all health care units now have infection control policies, therefore only the basic principles will be highlighted in this chapter.

It is recommended that all patients should be treated the same and regarded as a potential hazard, that is universal precautions should be used, as it is impossible to tell who is infected with HIV, hepatitis B or other blood-borne infections (RCN, 1994). Barrier methods to prevent contamination by blood or bloodstained body fluids should be routine as good practice.

Pratt (1995) makes the following points with regard to universal precautions:

1. Handwashing should be carried out before and after patient contact, and all cuts and abrasions covered.
2. Gloves and aprons should be worn when handling body fluids, etc., or soiled equipment.
3. Masks and eyewear should be worn during procedures that may cause droplets to be generated or when there is heavy contamination of the environment with blood or body fluids.
4. If hands are contaminated, they should be washed immediately with an antiseptic solution.
5. Needles must not be resheathed and safe, effective sharps disposal is paramount.
6. Biohazard labels on specimens from HIV-positive patients may still be required under local policy, though the use of universal precautions should make this unnecessary.

The RCN (1994) recommend that all blood spillage is treated with a chlorine-releasing agent before being cleaned with gloved hands and then washed.

Needlestick injuries

Although health care workers are at risk of being infected with blood-borne infections including HIV, the occupational risk of becoming infected with HIV is dependent on the prevalence of infection within the work area (Parker, 1992).

The estimated risk of seroconversion after a needlestick injury (percutaneous transmission) with HIV-infected sharps has been quantified by Heptonstall, Porter and Gill (1995) as being 0.32% and Ingram (1993) notes that it is thought that at least 0.1 ml of blood infected with HIV is needed for infection to occur as a result of a needlestick injury, in contrast to hepatitis B infection, which requires only 0.00004 ml of blood. One reported case of a nurse being infected with HIV occurred when an intravenous cannula introducer was jabbed into her arm following resuscitation of an HIV-positive patient (Eaton, 1993). Heptonstall, Porter and Gill (1995) also note a 0.03% seroconversion rate after mucocutaneous (through mucosa or skin) exposure to HIV occupationally.

It is important that all nurses working in GUM are aware of their local policy in relation to needlestick injury. The policy of the working area of one of the authors states that the following points should be considered (Glan Hafren NHS Trust, 1994):

- occupational health or GUM clinic should be contacted;
- advice on avoiding possible transmission, e.g. protected sexual intercourse, avoiding getting pregnant, should be given;
- zidovudine prophylaxis should be considered;
- blood should be taken from the health care worker for HIV testing and storage and from the source patient if consent is given;
- follow-up and support should include blood tests at 6 weeks, 3 months and 6 months.

The RCN (1994) advises that penetrating injuries should be made to bleed, washed thoroughly with soap and running water and then covered with a waterproof plaster. It is also important to remember not to suck the wound.

Routine monitoring of patients

Routine monitoring of patients with HIV infection varies from clinic to clinic, as does the frequency of appointments, but nurses in GUM are likely to be involved in taking specimens of blood, etc. and should be prepared to answer patients' questions on the tests being taken.

A full physical examination is normally made, checking the heart, lungs, condition of the skin, eyes, ears and mouth. Reflexes and sensation are tested and temperature, pulse, blood pressure, weight and oxygen saturation are monitored and routine urinalysis is done. If the patient has signs or symptoms of infection, a throat swab, sputum specimens, faeces specimens, midstream urine or blood cultures might be taken. Women should have regular cervical cytology.

Patients may have urine tested for neopterin and creatinine levels as indicators of disease progression (Squire & Johnson, 1992). A full blood count is taken including erythrocyte sedimentation rate (ESR), as various haematological changes may be seen including a slight reduction in haemoglobin level, reduced platelet count, a raised ESR and a low lymphocyte count, particularly the CD4 count (Gilson, 1996). Urea and electrolytes and liver function tests are taken regularly, particularly when a patient is on any treatment, as so many of the drugs given are toxic to the liver and kidneys. CD4 and CD8 lymphoctye counts are taken to monitor progression of disease and a patient whose CD4 count has dropped to $200 \times 10^6/1$ or below is considered to be at risk of developing severe opportunistic infections (Gilson, 1996). A rise in beta-2-microglobulin (B^2 microglobulin) levels is also believed to be a marker for disease progression and this level is generally monitored regularly (Squire & Johnson, 1992). Pratt (1995) notes that a rise in p24 antigen is a marker for progression to symptomatic illness and p24 level is generally monitored.

When patients are first diagnosed they will have baseline tests for infections such as cytomegalovirus and toxoplasmosis, as these opportunistic infections may be reactivated in symptomatic disease; also syphilis serology and hepatitis B screening are undertaken and gay men who are hepatitis B negative may be vaccinated (Gilson, 1996).

Drugs used in HIV disease

A large number of drugs are used in treating HIV-positive patients because of the wide range of individual infections and symptoms that may occur, therefore only a few of the commonest drugs given as outpatient treatment will be discussed here.

Candidal infection of the mouth, oesophagus, vagina and perianal area is often seen in patients with HIV and is generally treated with systemic drugs. Mindel (1996) suggests ketoconazole 200–400 mg daily for 10–14 days or fluconazole 50–100 mg daily for 10–14 days, though some patients will need repeated courses or higher doses, up to 400 mg of fluconazole, if they do not show a good response. Clotrimazole vaginally may be given for vulvovaginal candidiasis, though oral treatments may be needed (Pratt, 1995).

Aciclovir 200 mg four times a day or aciclovir 5% ointment 6-hourly may be given for recurrent *Herpes simplex* virus infection, as lesions can be very troublesome around the mouth in some patients (Zakrzewska, 1996).

Once the CD4 level is $200 \times 10^9/1$ or below, most physicians start asymptomatic patients, or earlier in symptomatic disease, on prophylaxis for *Pneumocystis carinii* pneumonia (PCP), either oral co-trimoxazole (Septrin) 960 mg daily or, if this is not tolerated, nebulised pentamidine 300 mg monthly (Miller, 1996). GUM nurses must be aware of the precautions needed with pentamidine if they are involved in its administration, namely that it should only be given in a room with external ventilation (Pratt, 1995). The manufacturers note that pregnant staff should not be involved in caring for patients having nebulised pentamidine, as it may damage the foetus; nurses should remain outside the room while this treatment is in progress and wear a high filtration mask if they must enter the room; and nurses with asthma should avoid caring for patients having this treatment, if possible (May & Baker, 1994).

Antiviral therapy

Patients may be offered various antiviral drugs, which work by interfering with the process of virus replication by inhibiting the action of reverse transcriptase. The first drug to be used was zidovudine (Retrovir), formerly known as AZT, and patients are generally prescribed a dose of 500–600 mg daily (Pratt, 1995). Pratt also discusses the use of newer drugs with similar actions, didanosine (ddI) and zalcitabine (ddC), which are also licensed for use, and stavudine (d4T), 3TC and PMEA, all of which are undergoing clinical trials at present.

Recent research and ongoing trials have shown that combination therapy, often zidovudine with either didanosine or zalcitabine, seems to give longer-lasting activity against HIV than zidovudine on its own (monotherapy) and combination therapy is now routine (Williams & Weller, 1996).

These drugs can have very toxic side effects and there is much ongoing research and debate about their use, including at what stage in the disease progression they should be given. Patients may be very well-informed about drug trials and treatments and nurses should keep up-to-date with new developments, as well as the moral and ethical dilemmas of such treatments.

Continuing care, rehabilitation and complementary therapy

In many GUM clinics, there is close liaison between clinic nurses and community nurses to enhance the continuing care of patients. Nursing models and documentation may be used to ease the transition process and Griffiths-Jones and Walker (1993) describe the use of Roy's adaptation model in HIV care. They believe this model of care gives nurses and patients a good understanding of stress factors and coping mechanisms employed by the patient.

Worsley (1996) highlights that nurses caring for patients with HIV and AIDS need to work collaboratively with both patients and the multidisciplinary team, to allow development in care, and that some nurses find the patient-led approach to HIV care difficult to cope with. It is important, therefore, that GUM nurses critically evaluate their practice, to ensure quality nursing care is provided for people infected or affected by HIV (Hicken & Faugier, 1996b).

Part of a quality service is providing rehabilitation for HIV patients, as described by Wells (1993). He suggested that the needs of patients with AIDS should be met by a holistic approach based on rehabilitation, and nurses should not see rehabilitation as something that happens at too late a stage, when doctors are unable to do anything further.

The RCN (1994) suggests that complementary therapies may be of great benefit to HIV-positive patients by enhancing care and quality of life, often in tandem with conventional medical treatment and rehabilitation. They suggest that complementary therapies can help in reducing anxiety and stress, while improving general wellbeing; they can help with sleeping problems and pain control as well as helping patients who are trying to reduce or stop drug or alcohol consumption. Sofroniou (1993) notes that some practitioners believe that aromatherapy oils and massage can help patients with HIV and AIDS by giving a sense of wellbeing and reducing the feeling of being an outcast through the use of touch, and certain oils, such as tea-tree, can help to boost the immune system. In addition, complementary therapies can also be of help to staff who may be under great stress when caring for patients with HIV and AIDS (RCN, 1994).

Bereavement counselling in HIV disease

The RCN (1994) suggests that grief associated with HIV infection starts for the patient when the diagnosis is given. As a result, GUM nurses have a special role in bereavement counselling with the patient, their partners and carers. Miller et al. (1993) suggest that the reversal of life expectancy and quality of life in young people with HIV is an important aspect and that HIV may also reverse the natural cycle of parents dying before their children, which parents may find very difficult to accept and deal with.

Although much of the terminal-stage counselling and bereavement counselling of significant others may occur in the community or be given by specialist counsellors, GUM nurses should be aware of the processes involved in grief, as well as understanding that patients may wish to talk, as HIV infection can lead to isolation from family and friends, and stigma and prejudice on the part of others (RCN, 1994). The stigma and secrecy that are part of HIV mean that nurses may have to deal with issues of confidentiality at the time of or after the patient's death and also play a key role in helping the medical team and the patient's carers to communicate (Miller et al., 1993).

Allowing a patient to put their affairs in order, including planning the funeral, may be stressful for nurses but is part of the counselling process (RCN, 1994). Miller et al. (1993) note that nurses must find effective approaches in bereavement counselling and also recognise when specialist bereavement counselling from those with further training and experience is needed.

Living wills and advanced directives

Living wills do not have any legal standing in the UK at present and both the British Medical Association and the RCN have rejected the idea of legalising living wills, though they advise that account should be taken of a patient's wish expressed in a living will (Wright, 1996). The RCN (1994) notes that advanced directives or living wills allow patients with HIV and AIDS to take control over their illness and death and that patients may appoint someone as a proxy to act for them, if they are unable to do so. Cowe (1996) believes that nurses can help honour the patient's wishes if they accept the use of living wills, even when they do not agree with the patient's wishes, though education and clarification of the role of nurses in relation to living wills are needed. Nurses in GUM should be aware of their patients' wishes and know if living wills have been made, to allow holistic care of patients up to death.

Clinical supervision for nurses

Nurses in GUM may find that they are unable to discuss the problems of death, sex and contagion and the stigma of HIV with their colleagues, though they may be heavily involved with or affected by HIV due to the nature of the close relationship with their patients (Palmer, 1995). As a result, nurses may have differing needs for support, relating to lack of knowledge, attitudes or the emotional stress of looking after seriously ill young people, and clinical supervision has the potential to meet these needs.

The RCN (1994) suggests that a formal arrangement for supervision and support may help protect against burnout in staff. This is endorsed by Faugier and Hicken (1996b), who believe that effective clinical supervision can help nurses to channel their commitment and energy to the benefit of their own self-esteem and the best interests of their patients. As Lempp (1995) notes, burnout for nurses working with HIV and AIDS patients needs to be reduced by supportive programmes and environments, and teamwork is a key to this. Therefore, GUM nurses should advance their role as part of a multidisciplinary team to enhance patient care and continue their own professional development.

Networking

It is important that nurses in GUM work with other agencies for the benefit of HIV-positive patients and to this end, they should know how patients can access local and national support services such as Body Positive, Terrence Higgins Trust, Positively Women, Mainliners, and local HIV and drug support groups. Many of these addresses are given at the end of Chapter 3. Below are some of the groups and people that GUM nurses may need to network with:

- health visitors for children;
- midwives;
- community nursing staff;
- physiotherapists;
- dietitians;

- chiropodists;
- community psychiatric nurses dealing with patients with drug problems and patients with dementia;
- local schools and colleges and health education departments;
- other health authorities and trusts;
- social services and benefits officers;
- consultants and GPs;
- clergy;
- local support groups;
- local AIDS advisory groups and RCN AIDS Forum representatives;
- the Genito-Urinary Nurses Association (GUNA).

Conclusion

Hicken and Faugier (1996a) quote Richard Wells' words: 'If we can get it right for people with AIDS then we will get it right for everyone else'. This is the challenge ahead for GUM nurses, in all aspects of sexual health nursing.

References

Akinsanya JA, Rouse P (1992) Who will care? A survey of the knowledge and attitudes of hospital nurses to people with HIV/AIDS. Journal of Advanced Nursing 17: 400–1.

Bor R, Miller R, Goldman E (1992) Theory and Practice of HIV Counselling – A Systematic Approach. London: Cassell.

Cameron S, Wallis C, Blakely A (1995) Setting up an HIV-testing service with same-day results. Nursing Times 91(40): 33–4.

Carlisle D (1995) No child's play. Nursing Times 91(43): 14–15.

CDSC (1996) AIDS and HIV-1 infection in the United Kingdom: monthly report. Communicable Disease Report 6(11): 99–100.

Cowe F (1996) Living wills: making patients' wishes known. Professional Nurse 11(6): 362–3.

Coyne P, Clancy C (1996) Out of sight, out of mind. In Faugier J, Hicken I (Eds), AIDS and HIV – The Nursing Response. London: Chapman & Hall.

Cranfield S (1996) Reducing inequality of access and care provision for people affected by HIV/AIDS. In Faugier J, Hicken I (Eds), AIDS and HIV – The Nursing Response. London: Chapman & Hall.

DOH (1993) The Health of the Nation: Key Area Handbook HIV/AIDS and Sexual Health. London: HMSO.

DOH (1995) Sexually Transmitted Diseases, England 1994. Department of Health Statistical Bulletin. London: HMSO.

Eaton L (1993) Double jeopardy. Nursing Times 89(19): 20.

Faugier J, Hicken I (1996a) HIV/AIDS research evidence – dilemmas and lessons in a multiprofessional context. In Faugier J, Hicken I (Eds), AIDS and HIV – The Nursing Response. London: Chapman & Hall.

Faugier J, Hicken I (1996b) Clinical supervision and staff support in HIV and AIDS nursing. In Faugier J, Hicken I (Eds), AIDS and HIV – The Nursing Response. London: Chapman & Hall.

Firn S, Norman IJ (1995a) Pyschological and emotional impact of an HIV diagnosis. Nursing Times 91(8): 37–9.

Firn S, Norman IJ (1995b) Nurses' role in supporting people who are HIV positive. Nursing Times 91(12): 37–9.

Friend B (1992) Invisible women. Nursing Times 88(49): 18.

Gilson RJC (1996) Early HIV infection – clinical features and management. In Mindel A, Miller R (Eds), AIDS – A Pocket Book of Diagnosis and Management, 2nd edn. London: Arnold.

Glan Hafren NHS Trust (1994) Management of an Outbreak of Infectious Diseases at Hospitals within the Glan Hafren NHS Trust involving Patients and Staff. Wales: Glan Hafren NHS Trust.

Green J (1989) Post-test counselling. In Green J, McCreaner A (Eds), Counselling in HIV Infection and AIDS. Oxford: Blackwell Scientific Publications.

Griffiths-Jones A, Walker G (1993) A new way forward. Nursing Times 89(19): 76–8.

Heptonstall J, Porter K, Gill ON (1995) Occupational Transmission of HIV. PHLS internal report (unpublished).

Hicken I, Faugier J (1996a) Establishing a nursing agenda for HIV/AIDS. In Faugier J, Hicken I (Eds), AIDS and HIV – The Nursing Response. London: Chapman & Hall.

Hicken I, Faugier J (1996b) Strategic planning in the era of AIDS. In Faugier J, Hicken I (Eds), AIDS and HIV – The Nursing Response. London: Chapman & Hall.

Ho DD, Neumann AU, Perelson AS, Chen W, Leonard JM, Markowitz M (1995) Rapid turnover of plasma virions and CD4 lymphocytes in HIV-1 infection. Nature 373(6510): 123–6.

Illman J (1993) History lesson. Nursing Times 89(26): 26–9.

Ingram J (1993) Avoiding the risk of needlestick injuries. Nursing Standard 7(17): 25–8.

Lempp H (1995) Burnout associated with caring for people living with HIV/AIDS. Nursing Times 91(18): 34–5.

Lineham T (1993) Barred from safe sex. Nursing Times 89(12): 16–17.

Loveday C (1996) Virology of AIDS. In Mindel A, Miller R (Eds), AIDS – A Pocket Book of Diagnosis and Management, 2nd edn. London: Arnold.

Mackereth P, Harrison T (1995) Maintaining confidentiality when tracing contacts. Nursing Times 91(2): 25–6.

May & Baker (1994) Pentacarinat ready-to-use solution. Drug Information Leaflet. Dagenham: May & Baker.

McCreaner A (1989) Pre-test counselling. In Green J, McCreaner A (Eds), Counselling in HIV Infection and AIDS. Oxford: Blackwell Scientific Publications.

Miller R (1996) Respiratory manifestations of AIDS. In Mindel A, Miller R (Eds), AIDS – A Pocket Book of Diagnosis and Management, 2nd edn. London: Arnold.

Miller R, Bor R, Goldman E, Ormanese M, Harvey V (1993) Bereavement counselling in HIV disease. Nursing Standard 7(39): 48–51.

Mindel A (1996) Gastrointestinal and miscellaneous clinical problems. In Mindel A, Miller R (Eds), AIDS – A Pocket Book of Diagnosis and Management, 2nd edn. London: Arnold.

Mortimer PP (1993) The 'AIDS' virus and the HIV test. Medicine International 21(1): 19–24.

Murray J, Johnson AM (1996) AIDS – epidemiology and natural history. In Mindel A, Miller R (Eds), AIDS – A Pocket Book of Diagnosis and Management, 2nd edn. London: Arnold.

Palmer H (1995) Clinical supervision for nurses working with people with HIV/AIDS. Professional Nurse 11(10): 20–2.

Parker L (1992) For safety's sake. Nursing Times 88(45): 56–8.

Plant F (1995) Unseen and unheard. Nursing Times 91(24): 17.

Platzer H (1993) Nursing care of gay and lesbian patients. Nursing Standard 7(17): 34–7.

Pratt R (1995) HIV and AIDS – A Strategy for Nursing Care, 4th edn. London: Edward Arnold.

Rees J (1995) The family way. Nursing Times 91(20): 48–9.

Rowe E (1994) A sexual health service for male sex-industry workers. Nursing Times 90(27): 42–3.

Royal College of Nursing HIV Nursing Society (1994) AIDS/HIV Infection Nursing Guidelines, 2nd edn. London: RCN.

Singh S (1994) A medical perspective. In Cusack L, Singh S (Eds), HIV and AIDS Care – Practical Approaches. London: Chapman & Hall.

Singh S, Cusack L (1994) Introduction. In Cusack L, Singh S (Eds), HIV and AIDS Care – Practical Approaches. London: Chapman & Hall.

Sofroniou P (1993) Aromatherapy. In Complementary Therapy. London: Nursing Times/Macmillan.

Squire SB, Johnson MA (1992) Medical aspects of HIV infection. In Theory and Practice of HIV Couselling: A Systematic Approach. London: Cassell.

Wei X, Ghosh SK, Taylor ME, Johnson VA, Emini EA, Deutsch P, Lifson JD, Bonhoeffer S, Nowak MA, Hahn BH, Saag MS, Shaw GM (1995) Viral dynamics in human immunodeficiency virus type 1 infection. Nature 373(6510): 117–22.

Wells R (1993) The rehabilitation of people with AIDS. Nursing Standard 7(25): 51–3.

Westcott P (1994) Women and AIDS. In Women's Health. London: Nursing Times/Macmillan.

Williams IG, Weller IVD (1996) Antiviral therapy and vaccines. In Mindel A, Miller R (Eds), AIDS – A Pocket Book of Diagnosis and Management, 2nd edn. London: Arnold.

Winship G (1995) Counselling drug users. Nursing Times. 91(20): 26–8.

World Health Organization (1995) AIDS global data. Weekly Epidemiological Record 27: 193–6.

Worsley MA (1996) Hospital services and HIV/AIDS. In Faugier J, Hicken I (Eds), AIDS and HIV – The Nursing Response. London: Chapman & Hall.

Wright S (1996) AIDS: ethical dilemmas and the nursing response. In Faugier J, Hicken I (Eds), AIDS and HIV – The Nursing Response. London: Chapman & Hall.

Zakrzewska JM (1996) Oral manifestations of HIV/AIDS. In Mindel A, Miller R (Eds), AIDS – A Pocket Book of Diagnosis and Management, 2nd edn. London: Arnold.

Index